AGAINST THE CURRENT

FOOTPRINTS SERIES
Suzanne Morton, Editor

The life stories of individual women and men who were participants in interesting events help nuance larger historical narratives, at times reinforcing those narratives, at other times contradicting them. The Footprints series introduces extraordinary Canadians, past and present, who have led fascinating and important lives at home and throughout the world.

The series includes primarily original manuscripts but may consider the English-language translation of works that have already appeared in another language. The editor of the series welcomes inquiries from authors. If you are in the process of completing a manuscript that you think might fit into the series, please contact her, care of McGill-Queen's University Press, 3430 McTavish Street, Montreal, QC H3A 1X9.

BLATANT INJUSTICE
THE STORY OF A JEWISH REFUGEE FROM NAZI GERMANY IMPRISONED IN BRITAIN AND CANADA DURING WORLD WAR II
Walter W. Igersheimer
Edited and with a foreword by Ian Darragh

AGAINST THE CURRENT
Boris Ragula
Memoirs

Against the Current

THE MEMOIRS OF BORIS RAGULA

As told to Dr Inge Sanmiya

McGILL-QUEEN'S UNIVERSITY PRESS · MONTREAL & KINGSTON · LONDON · ITHACA

ISBN 0-7735-2964-0

Legal deposit third quarter 2005
Bibliothèque nationale du Québec

Printed in Canada on acid-free paper that is 100% ancient forest free (100% post-consumer recycled), processed chlorine free

McGill-Queen's University Press acknowledges the support of the Canada Council for the Arts for our publishing program. We also acknowledge the financial support of the Government of Canada through the Book Publishing Industry Development Program (BPIDP) for our publishing activities.

Unless otherwise noted, illustrations and photographs used in this text derive from the private papers of Dr Boris Ragula.

LIBRARY AND ARCHIVES CANADA CATALOGUING IN PUBLICATION

Ragula, Boris, 1921–
Against the current : the memoirs of Boris Ragula / as told to Inge Sanmiya.
(Footprints)
Includes bibliographical references and index.
ISBN 0-7735-2964-0
I. Sanmiya, Inge Vibeke, 1951– II. Title. III. Series: Footprints (Montréal, Quebec)
R464.R33A3 2005 779'.961092'092 C2005-902128-4

Set in 10.5/14 Sabon with FF DIN
Book design and typesetting by zijn digital

For Ludmila

Contents

Acknowledgments

I would like to express my appreciation and thanks to a number of people whose help, patience, and guidance contributed to the completion of my memoirs. Certainly, my wife, Ludmila, and my staff deserve special mention. All of the staff in my medical practice demonstrated a high level of professionalism and compassion for the patients that filed through the office doors. Irene Rayew, who worked with me for many years when I practised medicine, also had the patience to transcribe many of my dictated notes. Lieutenant Colonel Richard G. Moore, a family friend and former patient, also lent me much-appreciated moral support as I wrangled with the task of putting my stories into an organized form. I must also mention Reverend Lloyd Cracknell. Although Lloyd and I often differed in our political views, we remained steadfast friends. Of course, my children, who saw little of me during the years that I worked to build my medical practice, have always given their heartfelt love. Many others have also played a large part in my personal and private life, and while there are too many to mention, I will always remember and cherish their friendship. Chuck Ruud and Inge Sanmiya provided the practical means for this project to take tangible form. Also, I would like to acknowledge the work of Harry Holme, a very talented photographer, who provided technical advice with the illustrations for this work. To these people, and countless others, I offer my thanks and gratitude.

Boris Ragula, MD
24 July 2004

Foreword

There are many improbable life stories still to be told by the men and women who, about six decades ago, survived World War II and clawed their way to safety out of the rubble of warfare and created for themselves new lives.

The author of this book is the late Dr Boris Ragula, a retired medical practitioner from London, Ontario. Dr Ragula was born in the territory that is now Belarus. At that time, Belarus was a part of Poland, and that made him a Polish citizen, but in 1939, Poland disappeared. The Belarusians were caught between two rapacious powers – the Nazi Germany of Adolf Hitler and the Soviet Russia of Joseph Stalin. As a result of the 1939 agreement between these two expansionist powers (the Molotov-Ribbentrop Pact), Belarus was incorporated into the Soviet Union along with other Polish territories.

Although a plaything of irresistible powers (and not for the first time in its history), Belarus had nurtured a group of young people who wished to see their country independent and who looked back to the short-lived Republic of Belarus of 1917–18 as a stirring example of beginning nationhood. One of these young people was Boris Ragula, who had no country that he could truly call his own. The Germans interned him because he had fought in the Polish army. Then, as an escaped POW who had returned home, he found himself within the boundaries of a Soviet state that considered him an enemy because of his Belarusian views. To resist his powerful foes, Boris Ragula could call upon little more than the traditional Belarusian characteristics of persistence and quiet resistance, along with a readiness to seize opportunities when he sensed them.

The challenges Boris Ragula met were immeasurable: he survived several German POW camps, endured imprisonment and interrogation by the Soviet NKVD, escaped to the West ahead of the advancing Red Army with the girl of his dreams, gained the support of Belgian Catholics and Pope Pius XII, earned a Belgian medical degree, and launched a Canadian medical career with only a smattering of English.

Had he been less of a risk taker, Boris Ragula could not have overcome the odds against his survival and success. He would have been overwhelmed by the obstacles he faced. But he remained fixed on his life's single aim, inspired by his doctor father and nurse mother: to practice medicine at a very high level. And so he lived a life dominated by his determination to advance towards that goal, however circuitously. Readers will be struck by how many people gave Dr Ragula a hand along the way, but they will also note how often he created his own opportunities. Most of all, they will learn about the great human lesson that binds together this life story: being helped inspires one to help others.

Charles A. Ruud
Professor of History Emeritus
University of Western Ontario

Editor's Note

When I began to assemble Boris Ragula's scattered notes and papers, I realized that his stories provide a unique insight into a time and place in history often overlooked or ignored. Stalin's reign of terror and World War II created political and social upheaval in Belarus and elsewhere in Europe. Despite these obstacles Boris continued his struggle to achieve his lifelong ambition of becoming a medical doctor.

After the war Boris and his new bride, Ludmila, found refuge in Belgium. When he had completed his medical studies Boris embarked on yet another adventure, which brought him to London, Ontario. His determination, and the enduring support of his wife and family, played a large part in Boris's success as a family physician. However, what follows is not simply a story of personal achievement, but rather a critical observation of a rapidly changing world order. Furthermore, Boris's story exemplifies the difficulty of introducing new ideas and attitudes about healthy living into a complacent environment where personal security and freedom is all too frequently taken for granted. One of Boris's colleagues once referred to him as "a stampeding bull" that could not be tethered. Boris never apologized for the strategies he employed to encourage people to stop smoking, lose weight, and enjoy their freedoms. He marvelled at the miracle of a newborn child, and he wept when all his medical knowledge and skills failed to save a young life.

My primary role throughout the past months has been that of a scribe. Boris and I spent many hours together, and on each occasion Boris had yet another story to tell about his life. I found that Boris possessed a great talent for storytelling but lacked the desire and patience to write. So he granted me the task of recording, analysing, organizing, and integrating his thoughts and ideas into a coherent work. It seemed appropriate to write the stories as Boris's personal account, but at times I expanded on his reflections in order to explain the historical significance and context of events or situations.

As the manuscript began to take form I was engaged by Boris's subtle and sly humour, his integrity, and his profound love of life. His children, grandchildren, and members of his extended family have heard some of his stories over the years. By example, and through his words and deeds, Boris has guided people to celebrate their strengths and skills and to share with others in the freedom to live fully.

Inge Sanmiya

AGAINST THE CURRENT

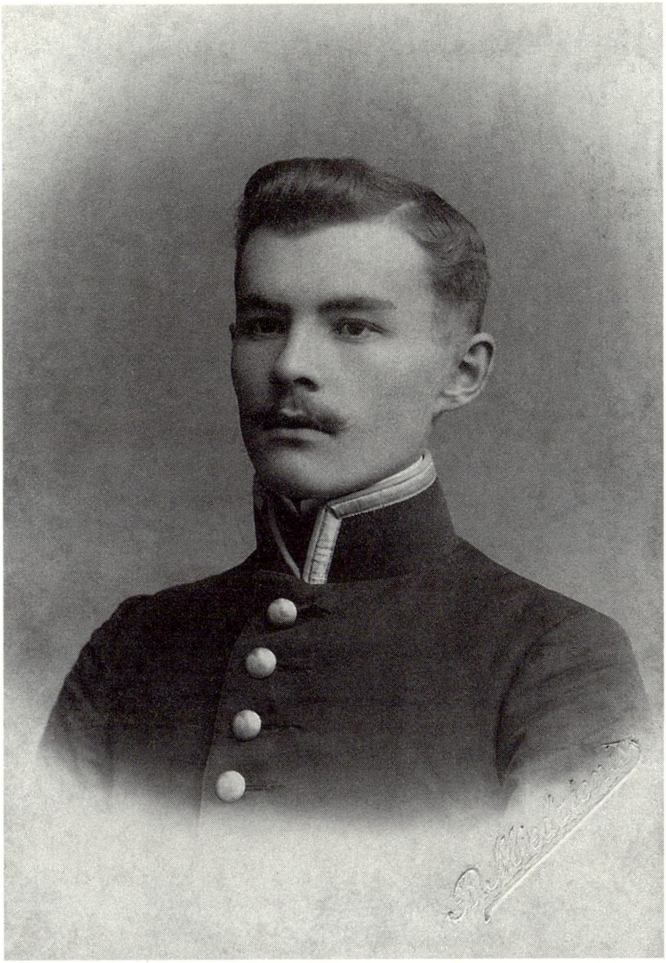

Dimitri Ragula, Boris's father, c. 1915, in the school uniform that he wore during graduation ceremonies marking the completion of his medical studies in Moscow

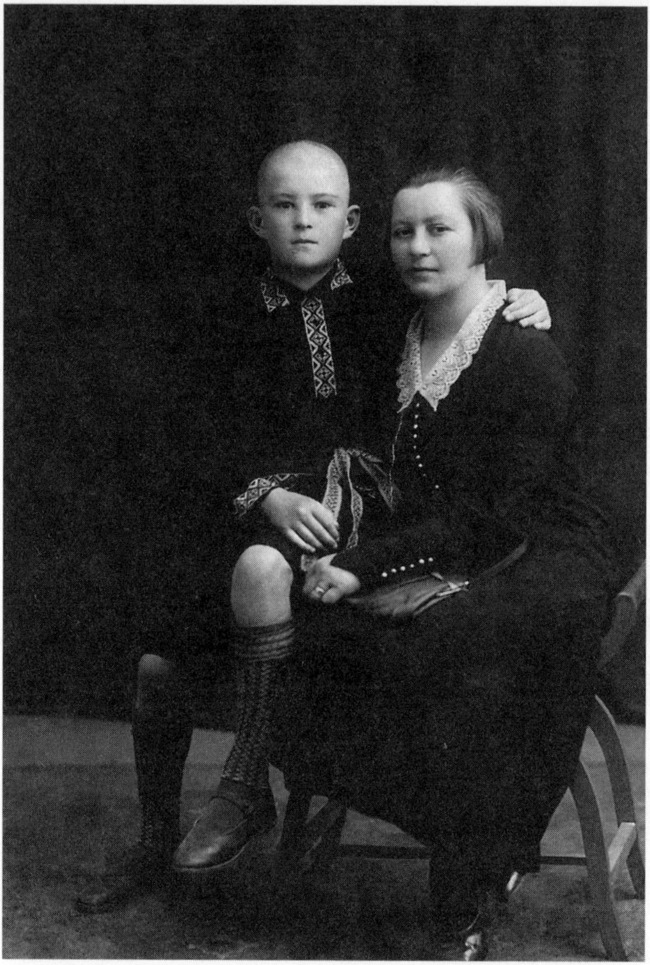

Boris and his mother, Nadzia, 1930

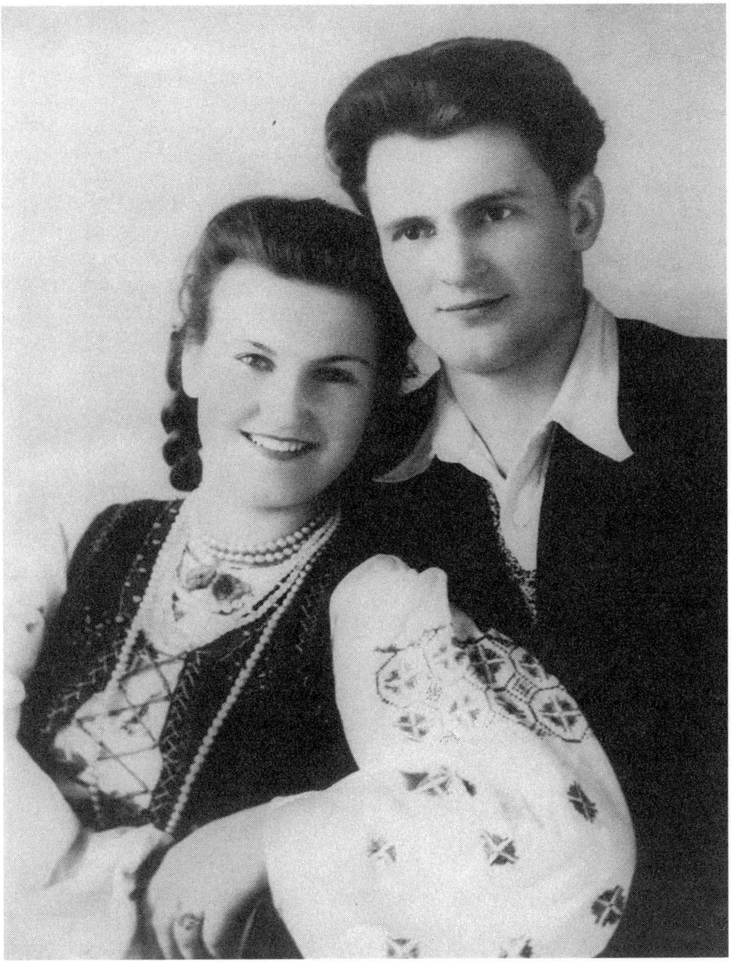

Ludmila and her brother Janka Hutor, c. 1940

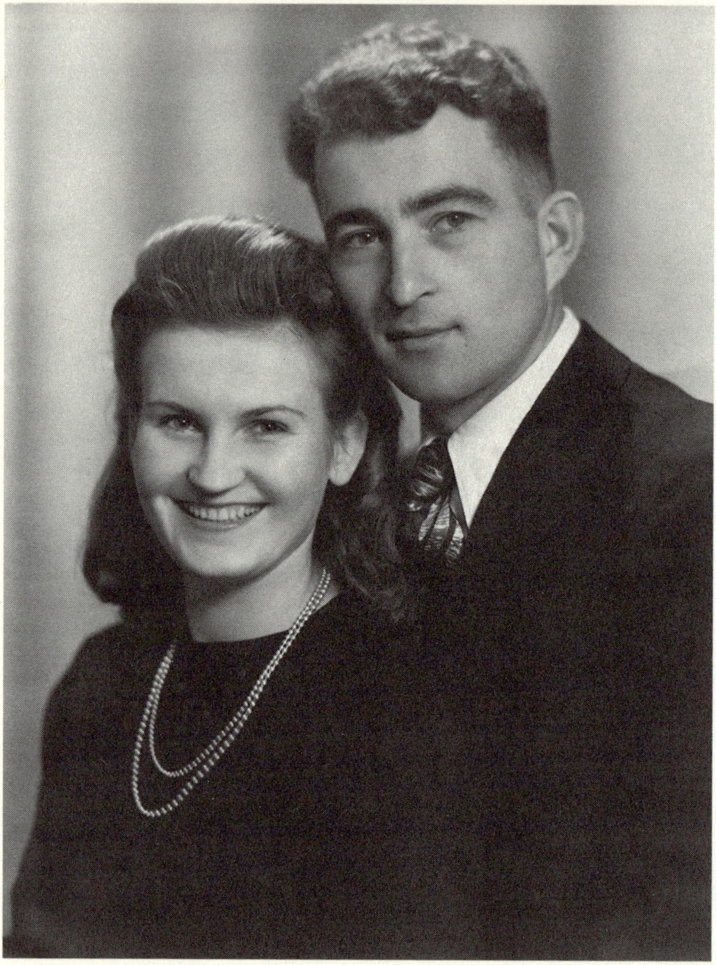

Ludmila and Boris, c. 1945

1 My Beginnings

In this book I will describe how I grew up, struggled, and survived in a country that remains largely misunderstood or overlooked in the annals of European cultural and regional history. In recounting my memories I have perhaps unintentionally distorted some events or circumstances that shaped my ideas and ideals, my hopes and my fears. Nonetheless, they are my memories, and they remind me that I made choices to live my life on my own terms. I also admit to an indulgence in nostalgic reverie, for I am eighty-three years old; yet much of what I experienced remains vibrant and alive in my heart and in my spirit. This book is also a story about new beginnings. At the end of World War II, with nothing to sustain us except blind, youthful hope and our love for one another, my wife, Ludmila, and I left Belarus. Some years later, after I had earned my medical degree, hope and love also gave us the strength to leave Western Europe and begin a new life in Canada.

While I realize that I have not played a great role in shaping international politics, I do lay claim to an enduring political activism and a passionate belief in human rights. Before I begin to tell my story, I want to outline briefly the history of Belarus, my homeland. The country's origins can be traced to Kievan Russia, the first East Slavic state to emerge in the late ninth century. After the death of its ruler, Prince Yaroslav the Wise, in 1054, Kievan Russia split into a number of principalities, each with a central city. Polotsk, located 120 miles northeast of Minsk, became the nucleus of modern-day Belarus.[1] The country has suffered, and continues to suffer, devastating political, economic, and cultural hardships brought about by the nationalistic and territorial ambitions of neighbouring states.

After the Tatar overthrow of Kiev in 1204 Belarus and part of the Ukraine came under the control of Lithuania. The resulting state was called the Grand Duchy of Lithuania. For a short time Belarusian culture flourished under this regime. The Union of Krewo (1385) joined Poland and the Grand Duchy in a confederation. This union hinged on Lithuanian Grand Duke Jogaila's conversion to Roman Catholicism and his subsequent marriage to Queen Jadwiga of Poland.[2] He became sovereign of both states and was known as Wladyslaw II. When Roman Catholicism became the official religion of Lithuania, the Lithuanian and Belarusian aristocracy converted from Orthodoxy to Catholicism and assimilated Polish culture, adopting the Polish language. As a result the Belarusian peasantry found themselves with rulers who shared neither their language nor their religion. Belarus remained a part of Poland until Russia, Prussia, and Austria carried out the three partitions of Poland in 1772, 1793, and 1795. After 1795, Belarus, with the exception of a small tract of land in the west, which fell to Prussia, became part of the Russian empire. Tsar Nicholas I (1825–55) endorsed a policy of Russification. The autocrat banned the name Belarus and replaced it with Northwest Territory. By the time serfdom was abolished in the Russian empire, in 1861, Belarus had been reduced to a nation of peasants and landlords. Although they had their freedom, the peasants had little else. The imposition of the Russian language, the Orthodox religion, heavy taxes, and mandatory military service (which lasted for twenty-five years) made the past under Polish rule seem benign.[3]

The outbreak of World War I, in 1914, turned Belarus into a zone of strict martial law, military operations, and unbelievable destruction. Large German and Russian armies fought fiercely and caused the expulsion of more than a million civilians. Russia's inept war efforts and ineffective economic policies created high food prices and shortages of goods and caused many needless deaths. Social unrest in the cities and the countryside led to strikes, riots, and the eventual downfall of the tsarist regime. Nationalistic Belarusians saw an opportunity to advance their cause during the period of disruption brought about by the two revolutions of 1917.[4] In December 1917 more than 1,900 delegates to the All-Belarusian Council (Rada) assembled in Minsk to establish a democratic republican government in Belarus. However, Bolshevik soldiers disbanded the Rada before it had finished its deliberations.

With the Treaty of Brest-Litovsk, which was signed in March 1918, most of Belarus fell under German control. Within a matter of days the central executive committee of the Rada nullified the treaty and proclaimed the independence of the Belarusian National Republic. Later that year the German government, which had guaranteed the new state's independence, collapsed. Belarusian Bolsheviks supported by the Bolshevik government in Moscow overran the new republic. By force of arms the Belarusian Soviet Socialist Republic (Belarusian SSR) came into existence on 1 January 1919. Belarus remained a political and territorial pawn during the Polish-Soviet War, a conflict settled by the Treaty of Riga in March 1921. Under the terms of the treaty, Belarus was once again divided into three parts: the western portion, which was absorbed by Poland; central Belarus, which formed the Belarusian SSR; and the eastern portion, which became part of Russia.

Belarus was under Polish control when I was born, in 1920, in Turec. My father, Dimitri, who had graduated from the University of Moscow in 1914–15, had a medical practice there. He had met my mother in Moscow while he was attending medical school and she was at teacher's college. The war separated them. Drafted by the Russian army, my father fought on the western front and my mother returned home to the village of Lubcza to live with her parents and two older sisters. While at the front my father was exposed to toxic gas, which earned him the medal of St Anne with Swords. This bravery commendation brought my father the title of nobility, but during the revolutions of 1917 all such nobility rankings were abolished. After the war my mother rejoined my father, but food shortages, hunger, and disease were widespread, and a typhoid outbreak decimated the Belarusian population. My father succumbed to the ravages of typhoid and died within a few short weeks. My mother found herself alone with no means to support me, a toddler of eighteen months, and my infant brother, Vladimir. Social and medical conditions continued to deteriorate, and soon after my father's death, diphtheria struck. Vladimir died a few months later.

With few alternatives open to her my mother again returned to her parents in Lubcza. Soon my aunt Luba and her husband, Konstantin Bitus, and their two children, Vladimir and Nina, came to live with us as well. My mother worked long days in the fields and tended the animals. Every Sunday she took me to my father's grave. I would stand quietly, watching her kneel beside the gravestone, and I would wonder what it would be like to call someone "Father." My mother would make the sign of the cross, and then we would walk the kilometre or so back home.

Although I have no real memory of my father I remember my mother speaking lovingly of him. She hoped that I would follow in his footsteps and become a doctor. I believe that this is why she kept his medical books, notes, and instruments. As a youngster I often looked at these articles, and I decided that my father had lived his life in order to help people. My mother and I shared a close bond, and she had a significant influence on the shaping of my values and ideas. Determined to become financially independent, she looked for work as a teacher, but although she had the qualifications, no one would hire her because she adhered to Belarusian Orthodoxy in a Polish Catholic district. So, with the reluctant consent of her parents, she enrolled in a Warsaw nursing school. My uncles Konstantin Bitus and Bazyl Ragula, the latter a senator in the Polish Parliament, promised to contribute to my mother's education. Aunt Luba also helped. My mother could not return home for holidays because travel was too expensive, and this meant that for the first time in my life I was without her.

I have many fond memories of my grandmother. She often slipped me special treats or came to my bedroom at night, rubbed my back soothingly, and recited prayers until I fell asleep. My recollections of my grandfather, Paul Oleszkiewscz, who was of Polish origin, are less flattering. He had an overbearing personality, possibly born of frustration and anger at losing his only son in an epidemic. He rarely showed kindness to his daughters and kept them subservient to his whims and desires. My mother's resolve to gain her independence must have been difficult for him to accept. As an Orthodox, he believed that the priest represented God himself. By contrast, my grandmother would regularly pray to different saints for different things. She explained to me that there was a saint for health, one for protection from lightning, one for protection from fire and drought, and even one to keep you prosperous. She believed that one should only address prayers to God when they concerned the most important matters. When I accompanied her to church, she would move from icon to icon, kissing each one and setting candles before them. She hoped that one day I would enter the priesthood.

When I was eight or nine years old my grandmother arranged for me to serve as an altar boy in the village church, which had a Russian priest who had come to Lubcza for his seminary training. We believed that he was a member of the Soviet Party. My observations and impressions of the priest and his brethren solidified my belief that Orthodoxy was a method of social control. I saw the priests collecting money and food from peasants who scarcely had enough for their own sustenance. Whatever the priests and their select circle of friends did not consume the pigs ate. When people went to confession the priests violated the sanctity of the ritual and reported supposed revolutionary activity or antigovernment sentiments to the secret police.[5] When I continued to speak the Belarusian language in the Russian Orthodox Church, the priest called me a filthy swine. I never went back to the church, but I continued in my own way to defy a system of repression that disgusted me.

During a celebration of Saint Ilya several priests and bishops arrived in Lubcza. Still smarting from the village priest's insults, I used threats and persuasion to convince the other altar boys not to dress for, or participate in, the ceremony. We watched the procession from the sidelines. Without altar boys the ceremony lacked pomp and splendour, and while this infuriated the village priest, it satisfied my rebellious spirit. When my grandmother discovered what I had done, she went to church every night to pray for forgiveness because I had "thrown an insult to God." She also told me that she would continue to love me anyway, but that I had committed blasphemy. I told her that I was sorry, but I could not accept the confines of the church.

My spiritual quest led me to find solace and peace on the banks of the Nieman River, the largest river in Belarus. There are many songs about this winding river, which meanders through the forest about two kilometres from Lubcza. I fished along the riverbanks, watched the sunrise, the flowing water, the birds. Here in this natural temple I could communicate with my god. I had no name for him, but I felt that he was a much higher power – one that could not be encountered in a church, for a church was too small to contain him.

When my mother graduated from nursing school she found work in Navahrudak and had accommodations in the hospital. I joined her there and started high school. Her talents earned her a promotion to head nurse in the operating theatres. She also worked as a midwife, assisting in home deliveries, and with her meagre hospital pay and the extra income from midwifery, we achieved financial stability and independence. Soon my mother had repaid my uncles, and she was able to give some financial assistance to her parents. Because we lived on the hospital grounds I was constantly exposed to medicine. Every once in awhile my mother would mention my father and express her hope that I, too, would one day become a medical doctor.

Each summer I returned to Lubcza, where I passed the long days with my cousins. We fished, explored the woodlands, and visited with relatives. I also helped my grandfather work in the fields and dig for bait. We would go fishing together on the Nieman River, and we often caught three or four pike and a string of perch. At nightfall we would set nets in the river, and early in the morning we would harvest our catch of whitefish, pike, and big catfish. A merchant living next door would hold some of the fish in his ice cellar for us so we could enjoy them for Sunday dinner, and occasionally Aunt Luba would prepare a Jewish dish of marinated fish. My cousins and I would sometimes sell our fish to buy sugar, which was an expensive commodity. The summers passed swiftly, and in September I would return to my mother in Navahrudak.

Polish authorities in Navahrudak had decreed that the Belarusian gymnasium had to enrol at least thirty-five students or close its doors. Teachers and students in the community had built this school with funds and materials donated by Belarusian peasants. In about 1932 two supporters of the Belarusian gymnasium, Mr Cienchanouski and Dr Orser, mounted a campaign to encourage parents and students to support the maintenance of the school. I was just twelve years old, but that did not prevent me from taking an active part. I spoke with friends and other young people and travelled to outlying farms to explain the situation. Once I had a heated discussion with a Belarusian student enrolled in the Polish gymnasium who insisted that the Polish school system offered him a better future, but I argued that he had no future as long as the Polish government suppressed Belarus. Despite this fellow's refusal to be swayed we finally managed to enrol forty-five students in the Belarusian gymnasium. Then the Polish authorities dealt us a bitter blow. They closed the school, fuelling the discontent and anti-Polish sentiments of many villagers. Students had the option of attending a Belarusian gymnasium in Vilnius or the Navahrudak Polish school. My mother, like other Belarusian parents, could not afford to send me to Vilnius. Ironically, my experiences in the Polish gymnasium strengthened my resolve to preserve my Belarusian heritage.

My friends Joe Sazyc, Vladmir Nabagiez, and Janka Hutor (who would become my brother-in-law), entered the Polish gymnasium with me. We felt like interlopers, and so we nursed our resentment and made few attempts to associate with the other students. Some were Jewish and Russian but most were the children of Polish settlers. The school authorities insisted that all students speak Polish, but our small group ignored this rule. Sometimes we sang Belarusian songs, which resulted in reprimands from the school director. When I insisted on speaking Belarusian in religion classes, the priest, with the approval of the school director, suspended me for two days. My mother protested, demanding that I and the other Belarusian students receive religious instruction in our own language. The priest continued to conduct the lessons in Polish, and in defiance we continued to speak Belarusian.

Our Latin teacher, unlike most of his colleagues, openly discussed the idea of national self-determination, giving examples from Roman and ancient history. The history teacher, however, was a different story – a Polish patriot who had earned a reputation for heroism while serving in the armed forces from 1918 to 1921, during the Bolshevik invasion. While I admired his bravery, I had no respect for his obvious animosity towards minority groups. I resented his perspective on the Grand Duchy of Lithuania, which differed greatly from Belarusian historical interpretations.

In the seventh grade – the equivalent of grade eleven in the Canadian system – this history teacher asked me to recite the words of the Polish anthem. I began, "Poland will never be lost as long as we are alive," but then I stopped, mindful of the hypocrisy I was uttering. I was not Polish. An uneasy silence fell over the classroom. The teacher stood in front of me with a stick in his hands. He suggested that I write the words on the blackboard. I stood my ground and gave him a cold, unwavering glare. He then suggested that I sing the anthem, and again I did not respond. I could feel the tension mounting, and I began to think that he would beat me with his stick. Instead, he broke the stick with his hands and ordered me to return to my seat. He never called on me in class again. I graduated with a C in history, which lowered my overall average, but I was still proud of it.

These experiences at school, as well as the stories told to me by my mother and other Belarusians about our cultural and political heritage, spawned my political activism. Close to our home there was a jail where the Polish authorities held Belarusians accused of harbouring Communist sympathies. The windows of the jail overlooked the hospital grounds. One day a stranger approached me and asked me to deliver messages from the prisoners: they would attach their messages to rocks and throw them from the windows; all I had to do was collect the messages and pass them along to the stranger. I readily agreed. Every morning before I headed off to school I would peer out of our apartment window and look for any sign of activity in the prison courtyard. If I saw a stone tossed from a barred prison window, I would retrieve the message and put it in my pocket. In the evening I would go to the village market to deliver the messages to the unknown gentleman. Soon I was enlisted to participate in other subversive activities and instructed to send messages to the prisoners. I would watch for a hand signal from a prison window, copy a coded message onto a board, and hold it up. If the communication had been successful, I would be informed with another hand signal. One day my mother returned home earlier than usual and caught me. I expected her to put an end to these communications, but she only begged me to be careful and told me that while she was proud of what I was doing, I had to remember that there would be official reprisals if the Polish authorities learned of my clandestine activities. For one thing, she could lose her position at the hospital. At my next meeting with the unknown Belarusian supporter, I explained my situation but agreed to deliver two more messages. My connection to this secret communications network ended, but my Belarusian patriotism had taken root.

Soon after this episode the authorities imprisoned my Uncle Bazyl, the senator in the Polish Parliament, for anti-Polish activities. I remember going with my mother to visit him in the prison. The guards searched my mother, but they ignored me. I had a message for my uncle, which I had concealed in my mouth, and when I kissed him I slipped the wad of paper into his mouth. The guards suspected nothing. After a short visit, we left quietly, and I could hardly contain my pride at executing such a plan.

According to the Polish authorities, all graduates of the gymnasium would be drafted into the reserve school of the Polish armed forces. Reserve school training lasted one year, and every year thereafter reservists had to do six weeks of retraining. The regulations also stipulated that graduates entering medical school would be exempt until they completed their study program, at which time they were required to enter the reserve school. After passing my final exams at the gymnasium I took special preparatory courses to upgrade my science credits. I planned to take my medical school examinations in Vilnius in late August and then attend Stefan Batory University. Only 100 out of 1,600 applicants were accepted to medical school, and only five placements were available to minorities, including Belarusians, Jews, Ukrainians, and Lithuanians. Imagine my exultation when I learned that I had been accepted. My mother and I danced around our small apartment. It was one of the happiest days of our lives. My friends Janka Hutor, Vsievolod Rodzko – whom we all called Vowa – and a fellow named Slawicki would also be joining me in Vilnius. Although Slawicki was Polish, we included him in our small circle of friends, and we enjoyed discussing everything with him – including politics.

But then my dream of attending medical school began to disintegrate. I received a letter from the armed forces notifying me that I had to begin my reserve training on 5 September 1938. When I showed my draft card to the dean of the medical school, he said that it was most probably a mistake and advised me to make preparations to enter medical school on 15 September. A few days after this meeting, the military police came to my home and ordered me to report to the reserve school. If I refused, they said, I would be charged with desertion. The same fate befell Vowa. We decided to go to the reserve school, explain our situation, and convince the authorities to grant us permission to continue with our studies. Our contacts at the medical school promised to do everything they could to keep our placements open until the issue was resolved. Nevertheless, we became reservists in the Polish army.

We soon learned what had gone wrong. Several influential Polish nationalists had intervened when they learned that three Belarusians had won coveted places at the university. I seethed inwardly, unable to accept the injustice of it. A few weeks later, the university notified me that another candidate would be taking my place. Later I came to realize that we could turn this predicament to our advantage – we could use our military training to further the cause of Belarusian political and cultural autonomy.

Throughout the training program Vowa and I applied ourselves to physical exercises, theoretical studies, strategy planning, topography, and cartography. I also began to have serious reservations about Vowa's emerging Polish sympathies. In a November issue of the reserve school journal, he published a poem celebrating 11 November as the day Poland had declared its independence. When I confronted him with this Vowa argued that he was trying to present an outward appearance of Polish patriotism in order to gain the trust of our oppressors. He reasoned that once he had attained a position of authority, he would be better able to aid Belarus. I grudgingly accepted his explanation, and he eventually proved to be sincere. Vowa would give his life for Belarusian freedom.

Political tensions in the country escalated. Since I had learned to speak German in high school, I understood the German radio broadcasts. I remember Hitler's March 1939 speech in which he demanded that Poland cede part of its territory to allow Germany access to the Baltic Sea. He wanted to build an expressway – an autobahn – through this territory and incorporate it into the German empire. This autobahn would link Germany with East Prussia and the Polish city of Danzig (the German name for Gdansk). Hitler assured his listeners that Poland would retain access to the Baltic, but should the Polish government mount any resistance to his expansionist plans, he would use force to achieve Germany's goals. Under the terms of the Munich Treaty, Germany had accepted Poland's political and territorial autonomy, but Hitler, with his twisted logic, argued that Germany was not invading Poland but merely exercising its right to connect the German people with East Prussia. The dictator's words carried a belligerent and threatening message. There were reports that Poland's foreign minister, General Joseph Beck, was refusing to grant Hitler's "request." Rumours circulated to the effect that German threats to force Poland to cede its territory were mere scare tactics because the German tanks were built of cardboard.

During discussions with my friends I argued that the Germans would not occupy the Rhine region, which had been demilitarized after World War I. I also asserted that Germany lacked the military power to occupy the Sudetenland. I believed that England would take steps to prevent Hitler from pursuing his policy of territorial expansion. However, the world soon learned that Germany did have the military resources and the political will to follow through with these plans. Initially, no one wanted to believe it. In an attempt to bolster public confidence, the Polish propaganda machine built a cult following for Polish leader General Edward Smigly-Rydz. Songs about Smigly-Rydz leading the powerful Polish nation to victory in Czechoslovakia proliferated.

During this time of uncertainty the reserve school cancelled all leaves, but I received special permission to return to Navahrudak to visit my mother, who had been injured when a Polish bomber crashed into the hospital. I yearned to see her. On the long train ride home, I tried to push aside my fears for her health and safety and concentrated instead on her warmth, her friendship, and her faith in me. Finally the train pulled into Navahrudak station, and I rushed to the hospital. To my great relief, she was sitting up in her hospital bed. Bandages covered her head and one eye, and she had burns on her hands and face, but all that mattered to me was that she was alive. My three-day furlough flew by. When I said my goodbyes I had no way of knowing that I would be gone for a long, long time.

In June 1939 I graduated from the reserve school with the rank of sergeant. Soon after graduation the military authorities assigned me to the Forty-second Regiment stationed in Belostock, a city considered by many Belarusians to be home territory. In late August I joined my platoon. Since there was no lieutenant to lead us, I assumed the role of temporary commander. The next day orders came through that all sergeants from the reserve school would be promoted to the rank of lieutenant.

Preparing for war, the Polish army was in chaos. Troops lacked proper field gear, rations, ammunition, and efficient weapons. Our platoon had only three light machine guns, so we had to rely on old-fashioned rifles with bayonets. The magazines of these rifles held only five bullets, and reloading was required after each shot. Soldiers could eat their reserve rations only when the battalion chief gave the order to do so.

On 25 August 1939 the German minister of external affairs, Joachim von Ribbentrop, signed a non-aggression pact with the Soviet Union's commissar for foreign affairs, Vyacheslav Molotov. Under the terms of this agreement the Germans and the Soviets would partition Poland. The Germans sought control over the central-western region of Poland, and the Soviet Union claimed the western territories of both Belarus and Ukraine. Regular recruits had no knowledge of these negotiations. By listening to German radio broadcasts I learned that Germany was officially claiming that it sought peace and that this goal had been the basis for the non-aggression pact. I recalled Hitler's earlier tactic of announcing that Germany would forge ahead with its plan, regardless of existing treaties or agreements.

A year earlier, in 1938, the Germans had overrun the Sudetenland in Czechoslovakia. Polish troops had joined in the frenzy and reclaimed Zaolzie, a Czech district coveted by Polish imperialists. Consequently, I had no faith in the Munich Treaty and Germany's promise not to invade any other territories as long as England remained neutral. Prime Minister Neville Chamberlain's policy of appeasement merely solidified Hitler's future plans for territorial expansion. With the stroke of a pen Germany assumed control of the industrialized regions of Czechoslovakia, which specialized in the production of army vehicles, ammunition, and weaponry.

A week after the pact was signed, on a hot and humid night – 31 August 1939 – I was ordered to lead my platoon towards the East Prussian border, where we were to confront the German forces.

Only the rear battalions, which were digging trenches behind our line of defence, had the authority to order a retreat. My platoon members took up positions in a valley surrounded by hills at about 7 p.m. I had mixed feelings: fear, anticipation, and confusion. Here I was, a Belarusian, an unwelcome minority in Poland, fighting in the Polish armed forces. I shook off these thoughts and forced myself to lead my men the best way I knew how. I dispatched sentries to survey the German border area, but by midnight they had not returned. Restless and unsure, I walked along our lines. Troops on the line relied exclusively on voice or courier communications. Using a field radio I reported our situation to the battalions in the rear and then encouraged the men to get some rest. But, despite our weariness, sleep did not come.

At dawn the skies exploded. Artillery fell behind our lines and grenades rained down on the fields of the forward flank. Through my binoculars I saw the frightening roil of relentless bombs and started to tremble. A fellow soldier came to my side and offered me a cigarette to calm my nerves. He told me that the men looked to me for strength and that it was my duty to encourage them. Deep within my soul I found that strength.

Soon we saw the German lines advancing. Our light machine guns covered the field with crossfire. Light German fighter planes appeared on the horizon, striking our positions with deadly precision. After a short volley we lost the heavy machine gun on the right flank. Within an hour we had lost the second one, which left us with only three light guns and our inefficient rifles. I advanced to the front dugout position and continued to shoot until my ammunition ran out. Still we received no order to retreat. The Germans were closing in on us, and our only weapons were the bayonets attached to our rifles. Finally the order to retreat came through, and we received some cover from the Polish artillery on the rear lines. At around 2 p.m. the regiment's colonel arrived on horseback to assess our position. He ordered a counterattack and led the way by galloping towards the German lines. For some reason the Germans fell back. We maintained our position until nightfall, and then under cover of darkness we fell back. My men had spirit, but they were poorly equipped and fed. Nonetheless, we fought during the day and fell back after dark, always heading in the direction of Zambrow. As we neared our destination we lost contact with headquarters and were forced to rely on our own resources.

On the morning of 17 September the Germans surrounded my platoon, which had by that point lost twenty-three of its original sixty members. We surrendered. Screaming German soldiers ordered us to throw down our weapons and come forward. One of them hit me with the butt of his gun, and it felt like he had broken my arm. Then he ripped the binoculars from around my neck. His captain barked at him to back off and then informed us that we were now prisoners of war but would be treated in accordance with the Geneva Convention. He asked me my name, and when I told him that I was the platoon commander he wanted to know why I was continuing to fight for a lost cause. Something about taking an oath and my duty as a soldier tumbled out of my mouth. To my surprise, he shook my hand and offered me a cigarette. When he learned that I was a Belarusian national he asked me why I was fighting the Germans, who supported the Belarusian people. I had no answer.

We marched for endless hours and joined other groups of prisoners heading for East Prussia. After we crossed the border I marvelled at the prosperous farms, lush meadowlands, and orderly villages and remembered the Polish propaganda about Germany's poverty and unpreparedness for war. We, and so many others, had been duped.

One day we stopped in a potato field and baked some potatoes; another day the Germans brought in field kitchens and fed us soup and bread. I met up with one of my Belarusian colleagues from the Forty-second Regiment. A third fellow, a Pole, said that we three should stick together and pool our resources if we wanted to survive. After I managed to get an extra portion of soup to share among us this Polish "friend" declared that it was every man for himself and turned his back on us. I never saw him again, but the encounter taught me a lesson in trust, friendship, and the frailty of human nature.

A few days later we found ourselves installed in a prisoner of war camp known as Stalag 1A near Konigsberg, East Prussia, surrounded by double rows of barbed wire fencing and machine gun installations. In crowded barracks we slept on straw beds thrown on the floor. At noon, and again in the evening, we received our rations of half a loaf of bread, margarine, and watery soup. I befriended a man named Koscik, who had been studying in technical school when he was called up by the Polish army. Together we conceived of a plan to make our lives more bearable. Koscik etched the word "Omega" on my cheap watch, and I wandered through the camp trying to entice a gullible German to buy it. One German soldier seemed interested, and we started to bargain. I explained that it was my father's watch and it had great sentimental value to me. He offered me two loaves of bread and a pound of sausage, but I declined. When he countered with three loaves of bread and two pounds of sausage, I said, "What good are memories if I cannot survive to enjoy them?" The goods changed hands, and I learned another lesson about human values.

Some weeks later the Germans sent a contingent of prisoners, of which I was a part, to work on a farm in the village of Wiesendorf, approximately seventy-five kilometres south of Konigsberg. One old soldier, our guard Herman, communicated the rules through me because I spoke German. He told us to work hard and enjoy the relative freedom of farm work, adding that if we tried to escape life would not be so easy for us. At night Herman locked us into our barracks, an old house with straw on the floor for bedding. The farm family showed us unusual kindness, supplying us with some clean clothing. We still wore our old uniforms, but fortunately we did not have body lice. The farmer, whom I took to be about sixty years old, had a wife, a daughter named Helga, and two sons who had been drafted into the German army. I enjoyed working in the open air but found it difficult to handle the horses and the double plough. When the farmer saw me carving crooked furrows into his fields he gave me some instruction, and soon I was managing quite well. As I laboured I thought about those long-ago days when I had worked in farm fields with my mother and grandfather. And at the end of each work day, when Herman locked the door to our make-shift barracks, I would remember that I was not a free man.

One night Koscik and I decided to plan our escape. Since Koscik worked in the kitchen, he would be in charge of our food supply, and I would plan an escape route. We set the date for 20 November because we wanted to leave before the heavy winter snows fell. At night, in low whispers, we reviewed our plan and speculated about what it would be like to return to our homes and families. But then my appreciation for a lovely face prompted a swift change of plan.

Helga, the farmer's daughter, often brought us food while we worked in the fields. Although I tried to suppress any outward sign of interest, I could not deny a strong physical attraction to Helga. Her blue eyes, blond hair, and alluring figure tormented my reason and fed my sexual fantasies. One evening in November, while I was working by myself in one of the barns, Helga approached me. My eyes were riveted on her swaying hips. She stood facing me, her warm and inviting body close to mine. In a sultry voice she asked me what I was thinking. A shiver ran through me, but I croaked out words to the effect that I was nervous because if we were found together then I could easily be sent to the gallows. I mumbled a warning that she also risked humiliation and ostracism if it became known that she had consorted with a prisoner. Helga ignored my words, gave me a gentle push, and we were cocooned in a bed of hay. As much as I wanted her, I struggled to my feet and ran back to the barracks. Koscik found me in a corner, my face wet with tears of fear and humiliation. When I told him what had almost happened he said that he was worried that Helga would accuse me of rape, or worse, if only to satisfy her frustrations. I immediately understood the implications and agreed that we should make our escape the next night.

While we were working in the farmyard the next morning we saw two gendarmes speaking with our guard. The guard came over to Koscik and me and told us that we were being sent back to the POW camp. We both paled. My mind raced as I considered all kinds of explanations and scenarios. Had Helga reported me? Had someone learned of our escape plans? Would we be tried or shot when we returned to camp? Within hours we found ourselves back at Stalag 1A, and I sank into an overwhelming depression. After two days in the overcrowded barracks my body was crawling with lice. We were sent to a delousing station once a week, but the lice would return almost immediately. The physical discomfort and depression impaired my sleep. At night muddled images of my mother calling me to come home bled into distorted childhood memories. I fell into a pit of lethargy, I lost my appetite, and I avoided social contact with others. Several Polish officers and doctors at the local camp hospital asked me to join them in a game of bridge, but I had no interest. Such distractions could not lift my burden of despair.

At some point in November 1939 I rallied and began thinking again about escape. The faint hope of a successful escape also drew Koscik from his melancholy, and our planning took on a renewed urgency. We needed wire cutters, a compass, maps, and food. Koscik started creating "Omega" watches again. We enlisted volunteers to help us secure supplies and promised to include them in our escape plans, but because we failed to obtain wire cutters and maps, our project stalled.

Only fragmented reports about events in our homeland filtered through to us in Stalag 1A. We were unaware that on 17 September

1939, the Soviet Red Army had taken control of western Belarus and created the Belarusian Soviet Socialist Republic. Soon after the Soviet occupation, wealthy farmers were accused of exploiting the peasants in order to accumulate wealth and power, but this was a pretext created by the Soviets for sending thousands of peasant landowners to Siberia and launching a collective-farm program. Any resistance to this, especially from professionals or the intelligentsia, resulted in automatic exile to Siberia. We prisoners of war heard none of this – instead we received false reports that all schools had been reopened in Belarus and that students could go on to university. My dream of attending medical school was reawakened, and I now had a fierce desire to escape and return home.

Within the camp emissaries selected from among the prisoners collaborated with the Germans. They encouraged us to enlist as volunteers in the German army, which would entitle us to considerably more freedom. These turncoat tactics disgusted me, and I wanted no part in them, but I saw the opportunity to use the emissaries' preferential status for my own purposes. My friend and fellow prisoner Vowa enjoyed more freedom of movement than the rest of us, and he also seemed to have unfettered access to food and other supplies that would be necessary for our escape, so I asked him for help. He tried to convince me that our plan would only result in further hardship, and that if we returned to the Soviet-occupied territories we would not find the freedom we sought. Nevertheless, he brought us the supplies, maps, and other equipment we requested.

We set our escape day: 20 January 1940. Three days before this I developed a fever, and my temperature shot up. The camp doctors suspected pneumonia. Although my muscles ached and I suffered a blistering headache and burning eyes, I willed myself to get better. On 19 January my temperature dropped slightly, and this strengthened my resolve to move forward with the escape as planned. Koscik visited me in the camp hospital and advised me to postpone the escape, but I would not be deterred. That evening I played bridge with the doctors, and I sat at the card table struggling to hide my tangled thoughts and emotions. I played badly, and one of the doctors asked me if something was wrong. I offered a feeble answer about my health and my concerns for my family, and he did not press for further explanation, but it seemed to me that his eyes pierced my soul and detected my secret. In turmoil, I returned to my cot.

After breakfast the next morning I saw a camp guard speaking with my doctor. When he left the doctor told me that I had to report to the commandant's office. In order to alleviate my obvious discomfort, the doctor assured me that the guard had seemed very relaxed and friendly. Soon I found myself standing before the closed door to the commandant's office. I knocked tentatively, and on the order I entered the room to find not the commandant, but a lieutenant, an aide, and an emissary. The emissary, a man named Cannaceae, sat behind the desk, and under the watchful eyes of the German officers he spoke to me in Belarusian, assuring me that with my knowledge of the German language I could find a more pleasant position. My duties would be lighter, and I would have the freedom to travel. Choosing my words carefully, I told him that I needed a few days to think over this offer, but I added that lice and the daily drudgery of the prison regime disagreed with me. He seemed pleased with my response and instructed me to send a message through Vowa, who, he informed me, acted as a liaison. Only then did I understand how Vowa had managed to get us all the supplies we had asked for. I was flooded with a sense of betrayal and doubt. Had Vowa told the Germans of our escape plans? With a pounding heart, I left the commandant's office and returned to the hospital.

As the day dragged on, I tried to rest. When the doctor checked me later that afternoon, my temperature had fallen to 37.5. Supper arrived, and I forced myself to eat because I knew that this might be my last real meal if we did attempt the escape. The doctor gave me permission to visit my friends in the barracks at about 8:15 p.m., but he warned me that I had to be back before the 9 p.m. curfew. We stood facing one another, and when he shook my hand, I understood that he was aware of what I was doing and was giving me his tacit approval.

At the barracks Koscik and I packed a few belongings and waited until the lights went out. Outside, temperatures hovered at minus forty and the snow had drifted over a metre high. Our small company of five prisoners crept out of the barracks and scuttled past the guards to the first line of fencing. When I snapped the wire with the cutters I imagined that the noise boomed across the yard, alerting a patrol stationed a mere thirty metres away. But there was no response. Once we made it through the fences we intended to scale a small escarpment to the elevated railway track. From there we would race into a densely forested area and rendezvous at a crossroads some distance from the camp. But as soon as the last man had cleared the fences, there were shouts of "Halt! Halt!" followed by a volley of gunfire. As I reached the railway tracks, searchlights flooded the area and I heard the clatter of a machine gun. Bullets whistled by my head and ricocheted off the steel rails in a burst of sparks. Adrenaline pumping, I ran – for how long, I do not know. Finally, exhausted, I arrived at the rallying position, where I found all of my companions. Everyone had made it. We laughed and embraced one another, elated with relief. After we had taken our bearings with the compass I prodded the men to stay on the move. Three men, all good Catholics, first wanted to kneel in prayer. I yanked them to their feet and told them they could pray once we had crossed the border into Russia. We marched all through that bitter, wintry night and stopped shortly before 6 a.m. It had begun to snow, and we crouched under the boughs of fir trees, resting and eating our frozen rations. We hoped that the blanket of snow thrown over us by the winter winds would keep us well hidden.

We stayed in the woods until about midday. Our original plan entailed locating a deserted barn or some other shelter where we could warm ourselves and dry our clothes. Towards late afternoon we set off and again marched through the night. Where we found the stamina and energy, I will never know – perhaps fear propelled us forward. Just before dawn on the second day, we came to a big barn and entered through its open double doors. Surrounded by stable smells and sounds, we milked five of the cows and hungrily drank the frothy warm liquid. Then we burrowed deep into the hay stored in the loft. Sleep came quickly. I was awakened suddenly by voices. A group of farm girls and stable hands had come to do the morning milking and other chores. I heard one of the German milkmaids complain that some of the cows were not giving milk. There was the sound of feet clomping up the ladder, and soon the hayloft was filled with pitchfork-wielding stable hands. I froze where I lay – now, I thought, those Catholic prayers would be appropriate! Miraculously, our presence went undetected, and the stable crew left after completing their chores.

We waited until nightfall, left the sanctuary of the barn, and continued our march towards the Soviet border. Snow fell heavily. By daybreak we had not managed to find shelter, so we hunkered down by a small river, hoping that the drifting snow would conceal our tracks. Later that morning we heard a blast from a shotgun and then a German voice ordering us to get out from under the snowbank with our hands up. Someone had seen our footprints after all. Scrambling out of my snowy cavern, I saw a hunter standing about fifteen metres away, his gun pointed at us. I explained to him that we were prisoners of war who were just trying to get home, and we meant him no harm. But, I warned, if he stood in our way, we would fight him. Slowly, he lowered the gun and told us to move on, but first he cautioned us that we had landed in a well-populated farming area surrounded by villages and heavily used roads. As he turned away I prayed that he would not inform the authorities.

Unsettled and anxious, we returned to our places by the river and waited for nightfall.

Before we could set off again we heard a babble of angry voices. The next thing we knew, we were surrounded by farmers armed with scythes and pitchforks and several helmeted, rifle-carrying gendarmes. One of the gendarmes started to beat me. With all the authority I could muster I shouted that we were prisoners of war, captured in uniform, and therefore protected by the Geneva Convention. When I told him that he had to feed us and return us to the camp, the gendarme's commanding officer came forward and agreed that we had rights under the rules of warfare but that his men would search us for weapons. After conducting a cursory body search the gendarmes escorted us to the village jail and fed us bread and milk. Within an hour the village authorities had loaded us into a covered truck and sent us on our way.

At Stalag 1A Vowa managed to take me aside and ask for the compass and maps. I quickly slipped them into his pocket. Guards herded us into the commandant's office, where we were joined by a tall, slim officer with grey hair and intelligent-looking eyes. He was wearing a Wehrmacht (German armed forces) uniform. I was deeply relieved to note that no SS agents accompanied him. In a calm, well-modulated voice, he asked the leader of our group to step forward. As I made a move to do so Koscik blurted out that he was in charge. With a mild abruptness the commandant told us to stop playing hero games as it did not matter to him who had led the group. He only wanted to know how we had executed our escape. With as much dignity as I could summon I explained that I could not provide him with this information because it could jeopardize our next attempt.

The commandant smiled benignly and said that he, too, had escaped his captors during World War I. He understood our position, but we had lost. I brashly replied that despite this loss, we would never give up our efforts to gain our freedom. Blithely ignoring my attempt at bravado, the commandant announced that we would be penalized in accordance with camp regulations – we would go without food and perform four hours of exercise for two days. We would then be transferred to another camp in Germany. He dismissed us with a nod. In the prison yard, Vowa shook my hand and called us heroes, and at the barracks, the other prisoners gave us gifts of food and cigarettes. We spent the evening singing songs and talking about our escape. For a small space in time we forgot about the camp – the lice and the hunger – that defined our lives.

A few days later we packed up our meagre belongings and rode in the back of a locked truck to the train station. At the station gates I met the camp doctor and Vowa, and they wished me luck. Once again Vowa drew me aside and tried to convince me to work for the Germans. And once again I asserted my belief that to work for the Germans would be an act of surrender. I did not want to leave on bad terms, so I tried to console Vowa with the promise that I would always consider him a good friend. Perhaps we would meet again one day as free men.

Our train was delayed two hours, but by nightfall we had embarked upon our westward journey. After a dreary twelve hours or so we arrived in a town called Bocholt. I was unsure of our location, but I thought we were still in Germany. We were taken by transport truck to the camp, which was a duplicate of Stalag 1A, and there, in the commandant's office, guards checked our POW identification tags. I was number 5747.

The commandant wanted volunteers to work in the hospital, and I saw this as an opportunity to escape the mind-numbing routine of prison-camp life. I claimed to be a former medical student and was assigned the job of hospital sanitarian – a male nurse who assisted doctors by dressing wounds, giving injections, and performing other tasks. My new position meant that I could live at the hospital, sleep in a real bed, and escape the barracks scourge of lice and vermin.

Although I had to leave Koscik behind in the barracks I promised to take care of him whenever the opportunity presented itself.

On the first rounds the doctor asked me to change a dressing. The patient complained of pain, and the doctor instructed me to give him an injection of morphine. I struggled to remain calm as I frantically tried to recall how my mother had performed this routine task. With as much confidence as I could muster I inserted the syringe into the morphine bottle, drew up the required dose, aspirated the syringe, and, with clenched teeth, injected the patient's buttock. There! I had done it! After rounds the doctor told me that I could join the regular nursing staff and be in charge of food supplies. This delighted me because it gave me a chance to obtain extra food for Koscik and my other friends in the barracks. I soon discovered that hospital staff shared my opportunism.

After I had spent several days at the hospital the order sheet called for me to go to central supply and pick up food and materials for the sixty-five prisoners confined to the hospital. The Polish doctor in charge, who was under the supervision of a German doctor, told me to delay declaring patients dead so that we could continue requisitioning goods for them. Once or twice a week we collected the surplus food and, as promised, I gave a large portion to Koscik. With better food and proper rest I began to regain strength and vitality.

One evening in April Koscik brought up the subject of escape, and although I enjoyed my hospital work I was interested – escape remained a priority for me. I had learned that we were situated close to the Dutch border, but I knew that in order to plan an escape we needed a better sense of the surrounding area. Koscik heard that prisoners were being sent to work on farms and at other installations located outside the confines of the camp, and he came to tell me about it with a big smile on his face. A nearby monastery required skilled gardeners, and we hoped that our willingness to learn would compensate for our scant knowledge of gardening. When the commandant interviewed us for the position I spun a story about my father serving as head gardener for a big Polish estate. Gardening, I assured him, was ingrained in me.

The next morning, after taking my leave from the hospital, I clambered into a truck with Koscik and set out for the monastery. According to our rough calculations it lay about thirty kilometres from the Dutch border. A hooded monk, who introduced himself as Brother Joseph, met us and showed us about the grounds. We assured him that if he was displeased with our work, it would probably be due to that fact that our training and techniques were different from what he was used to; we promised to work well and adapt to his requirements. Brother Joseph seemed satisfied with this earnest outpouring. He showed us to our rooms and explained that he would not lock us in, but if we violated his trust, then the monastery would suffer unknown repercussions from the German authorities. Contritely, we told Bother Joseph that he had nothing to worry about. Although we ruined a few hedgerows with our unorthodox gardening methods (I did not know how to handle hedge clippers), Brother Joseph smiled benevolently and said that he'd keep us on anyway. Relieved, we started to plan our escape for mid-May.

With relative ease we acquired a map, a compass, and other necessities. By our rough reckoning a brisk walk under cover of nightfall would bring us to the Dutch border. As we continued to perform our chores around the monastery we began to notice increasing numbers of armed forces personnel in the area. One company took up quarters in the monastery, but we could only speculate as to why they were there. Perhaps the French and English were planning an attack. On the morning of 10 May 1940 we listened to a German radio broadcast in the monastery kitchen. Commentators spoke of Germany's effortless occupation of Holland. I could not believe that this westward aggression by the Germans could proceed without resistance. In the days that followed we also heard broadcasts about the capitulation of Belgium and the retreat of the English Expeditionary Corps. At first I refused to accept this news, but Brother Joseph confirmed that the Germans now controlled the northern part of France as well at the city of Paris.

We had to suspend our escape plans, but we hoped that another opportunity would present itself. In the middle of May agents with the German armed forces sought us out. One spoke of the benefits of joining the German forces, emphasizing that we would be able to work, wear civilian clothing, and carry a special permit identifying us as foreigners. We had heard these recruitment speeches in the past and were preparing to refuse when the agent explained that if we signed on, we would be transferred to a special POW camp in the Polish city of Thorn. Koscik and I exchanged glances. We accepted the terms, figuring that Thorn, although in Polish territory, afforded us a better strategic starting point for our escape.

In mid-June we arrived in Thorn, and from there we were transferred to a camp called Fort Herman von Salza. Unlike other POW camps this facility had massive fortifications and high walls. We found our quarters in the lower levels of the barracks. Many of the inmates were Polish, but we also encountered members of the British Expeditionary Corps and Belgian, French, and Dutch nationals. The British prisoners, unlike their Polish counterparts, received Red Cross packages from England containing chocolate, cigarettes, underwear, shaving soap, and many other luxuries. Now I regretted my decision to learn German instead of English.

For a few days Koscik and I studied the camp layout, trying to find a way to scale the high walls. It looked hopeless. I knew that many of the Red Cross packages contained clothing, so I tried to learn enough English to communicate with the British prisoners. It seemed like our only way to get civilian clothing, which we would need to make good our escape. I noted that the British prisoners had their own commanding officers, who operated as intermediaries between the prisoners and the German authorities. Summoning all the courage I had, I approached a British officer some weeks later and asked him to help us. He questioned me thoroughly, and

I convinced him of our determination to escape. He arranged an exchange of goods for civilian clothes and advised me to volunteer for work assignments outside the camp walls.

At the end of July German troops came to the camp looking for volunteers to clean toilets for them at their encampment. We told them that we would do it if they would give us extra food for performing such an unpleasant task. They replied that we would get extra food if we did a good job. And so Koscik and I added "toilet cleaner" to our wartime resumés, which also listed "gardener," "medical student," and "watch salesman." Five of us – Koscik and I, along with our three fellow Belarusian conspirators from Stalag 1A – were assigned to the toilet detail and taken to the German encampment. From there we could see the nearby Vistula River, lined with marshes and heavily overgrown lowlands. As the days passed we volunteered to do more jobs for the German troops, including cleaning floors, doing laundry, and shining boots – anything that would allow us to roam the camp freely. When Koscik and I returned to our prison barracks at the end of the day, we discussed the guards' movements and possible routes across the river. We set the date for 8 August, and after some consideration we invited our three fellow Belarusians to join us.

On the designated morning, wearing civilian clothes under our uniforms, we passed through the prison gates on our way to work at the German encampment. We had arranged to meet at a place on the riverbank at about four o'clock in the afternoon. In order to decrease the chance of being detected, our three compatriots would slip away separately, and Koscik and I would follow as soon as the guards had completed their circuit inspection. We waited for the right moment, slipped behind some bushes, shed our uniforms, crawled under the perimeter wire, and found ourselves on the road. Before we could get our bearings we saw two German corporals approaching the camp on their bicycles. As they passed us we lifted our hands in a "Heil Hitler!" salute. They returned the gesture and continued on their way. Then we heard the camp sirens wail behind us. We quickly waded into the bog at the river's edge and submerged ourselves with only our noses and mouths showing. I was afraid that the marsh would swallow us completely. Finally darkness settled, and we made our way to a clearing by the river and washed off our clothes. It was by now too late to rendezvous with our compatriots, so we were on our own.

We marched on until we spotted an isolated farm from which we took some hand tools and a sickle, slinging them over our shoulders. Now, to anyone passing us on the road we would look like itinerant labourers. At the next farm we asked for work, and the Polish farmer hired us to help with the harvest. Later in the day we met his daughter, a dazzling blond with sparkling blue eyes. We told her that we were prisoners of war trying to make our way to the Soviet border, and she advised us not to tell her father because he, and others in the area, feared punishment at the hands of the Germans. She also gave us the names of some villagers who might be able to assist us, including a man who could ferry us across the Vistula. After a short stint on this farm we headed off in search of the ferryman. With little difficulty we made it to the east side of the river, where we resumed our role as itinerant farmhands.

At another farm the farmer's eldest son warned us that the Germans had intensified their search for POWs and those involved in the Polish underground, and this reminded us that we were still a long way from freedom. He also described for us the general conditions in Poland under German occupation, explaining that the Germans had created a Polish provisional government with limited administrative authority in the cities and villages. However, there was no doubt that the powerful SS, in their black tunics, and the SA, in brown shirts, held Poland captive. Many patriotic Poles supported the well-organized resistance movement known as Krajowa Armja (AK). Any active members or associates of this organization risked being sent to a German concentration camp.

The farmer's son explained that many Polish nationals continued to believe that the English and Allied forces would prevail over the Nazi regime, but rumours were still rampant that the Germans would overrun England and crush any European power that interfered with their territorial or political goals. Koscik and I took heed of this information and proceeded with more caution.

We finally reached the outskirts of Warsaw, where a farmer gave us some food and allowed us to sleep in his barn. The next morning he came to us with a small bundle of supplies and a warning that the Soviets had discontinued the practice of exchanging prisoners. Crossing the border would not be an easy undertaking. We thanked him and promised that when Poland and Belarus were free, we would visit him and repay his kindness. We walked on for about thirty kilometres and then stopped on a hilltop, from which we could ascertain that we were near the border separating the German and Soviet armies. We could also see the border-crossing point, which was demarcated by a pair of ominous-looking towers situated about one hundred metres apart. By the early evening we had reached a small farm, and we took refuge in the barn. Two young sisters appeared and demanded to know what we were doing there. I explained that Koscik and I had escaped from a German POW camp and were trying to return to our homes in Belarus. The older of the two girls, Wanda, asked us detailed questions about our service in the Polish armed forces. We produced our POW identification badges, and this seemed to reassure her.

Wanda listened as we outlined our plan to cross the border, and then she warned us that if we were caught trying to enter the Soviet Union we would be imprisoned indefinitely in a camp situated in an isolated part of the country. She simply shrugged her shoulders when we insisted that this could not be true. Why would the Soviets treat their returning citizens so badly? We should keep acting as farm workers, advised Wanda – her father feared German reprisals and would force us to leave if he knew our true circumstances.

Moreover, she pointed out, when working in the fields we would have plenty of opportunity to watch the border patrols and work out a strategy for entering our homeland. She promised to tell her father that she had met two young farmhands willing to work for food and shelter, and then the sisters went back to the farmhouse.

At about eight o'clock that evening Wanda returned to the barn and told me that her father would like to see me. At the farmhouse she did most of the talking, but when her father asked me what we knew about harvesting and handling farm equipment, I explained that Koscik and I had come from farming families and were familiar with most farm operations. He agreed to hire us and said that we could sleep in the barn and take our meals in the house. I stayed to share a meal with him, but Wanda excused herself to take food to Koscik in the barn. She was gone for quite a while, and in the meantime I asked her sister, Zosia, to show me around the farm. After a leisurely tour we slowly made our way back to the barn. I paused at the entrance and started coughing rather loudly. Wanda emerged from the semi-darkness of the barn, hair tousled and cheeks flushed. I said a polite goodnight, and Zosia and Wanda headed for the house. I found Koscik lying on his back in the hay with a smile on his face. I did not question him, but an irrational jealousy nipped at me.

Early the next morning the farmer told me to hitch the horse and wagon. To my surprise, I could not do it – the tack was nothing like those I'd used in Belarus. I struggled with the task, and when I thought I had finally mastered the straps and girth, I stepped back. The farmer gave the horse a slap on the flank and it bolted off, leaving the wagon behind. Peering at me from beneath his bushy eyebrows, the farmer said sharply, "I thought you were a farmer's boy!" Humbled, I explained that the harness rig was different from the ones that we had used on our small family farm, and the farmer left it at that. I retrieved the horse, and the farmer gave me a quick hitching lesson.

We worked side by side for most of the day. During our brief breaks I asked the farmer about the guard towers and the border crossing. As Wanda had done, he told me that the border was closed and it would be very dangerous to attempt a crossing. He also said that a lot of Poles tried to cross into the Soviet Union in order to escape the Germans and that there would soon be a war between Germany and the Soviet Union. I kept my thoughts to myself and continued to work. I noticed a ploughed line running along beside a path that the German border patrols used about one hundred metres west of the border crossing. At regular intervals we saw patrols marching along the path, and several waved or greeted us pleasantly. Their relaxed attitude gave me hope that a border crossing was possible.

After supper on our second day I told Zosia and Wanda that we had to leave. Wanda said that she wanted us to stay for a few more days, and Koscik, obviously smitten by her, urged me to take more time to study the border area, but he failed to convince me. I said, "We leave tonight at ten o'clock." The girls prepared a bundle of supplies for us. Saying goodbye tugged at our hearts. Young Zosia timidly planted a kiss on my lips, and Koscik and Wanda lingered over their goodbyes.

By eleven o'clock Koscik and I were at the border. When the patrols passed we scrambled into the ploughed line beside the patrol path. Border patrols checked the ploughed line daily for signs of people attempting to cross to the Soviet side of this rudimentary boundary. In order to confuse the patrols, I told Koscik to walk backwards through the soft earth. If the patrols noticed our footprints, then they would, I hoped, be duped into thinking that someone had crossed into German-occupied territory from the Soviet side. We managed the crossing without mishap and then ran until we felt that our sides would burst. On that still night I fell to the ground and kissed the earth. This was my homeland, my country, and my people. We were back in Belarus!

2 Freedom?

We walked on, and at dawn we came to a farm. Our uneasy knock on the farmhouse door was answered by a terrified man who asked us what we wanted. When we briefly described our escape from the German POW camp and our long homeward trek, the farmer recoiled as if we were lepers. "You idiots!" he shouted. "Go back and return with the Germans to liberate us!" He raged on about the oppressive conditions imposed by the Soviet regime. Then, panic creeping into his voice, he demanded that we leave and forget that we had ever come to his farm because escape to the Soviet Union was no escape at all. He slammed the door.

Koscik and I stood on the doorstep, stunned with disbelief. We turned and walked away in silence. Eventually I suggested that we make our way to Belostock, where Koscik had family. Two days later we arrived at our destination confused, hungry, and tired. When Koscik's aunt opened her door to us, we saw fear and sadness drain the joy from her face. She quickly ushered us into the house, refusing to answer our questions and telling us to wait until Koscik's uncle returned. He worked in the city administration and had a better grasp of the political and social situation. Meanwhile, she fed us, prepared hot baths for us, and gave us clean clothing and shaving materials. We felt human again.

Koscik and his uncle embraced in a tearful reunion. Slowly, with a resigned shrug of his shoulders, the old man began to explain how the Soviet Union had "liberated" Belarus on 17 September 1939. The armed forces had invaded the country and decreed that Belarus was now part of the USSR. At first, he explained, Belarusians had hoped that their situation would improve under Soviet protection. Soviet authorities had organized a liberation plebiscite that had confirmed the union of the west with the east to form a republic. Then, with brutal expediency, they had denounced landowners and well-off farmers (*kulaks*) as "undesirable elements" and dispossessed them of their property and freedom. Most were sent to Siberia. Koscik asked about his parents, who were considered quite well off, and his uncle told him that a black carriage had arrived at his parents' home one evening, and they were never seen again. Koscik's father, like many others who had vanished, had done nothing that could be termed revolutionary. He had continued to work for the railway and to farm his lands. A profound heaviness descended upon us. This could not be happening.

Koscik's uncle gave me one hundred rubles and implored me to leave and forget that I had ever been in his house, forget that I had a friend called Koscik. When I looked into his eyes I saw fear. I agreed to leave immediately. Koscik and I had been through so much together, and we cherished our bonds of trust and friendship. We hugged each other, trying to stem the flow of tears. I feared we would never meet again.

I went to the train station, where I hid in a grain car rather than risk being seen in public. According to Koscik's uncle, the authorities regularly checked peoples' travel documents and passports, and without official papers or identification I was vulnerable. The train I was on eventually pulled out of Belostock, and at the town of Baranovichi I disembarked and bought a ticket to Navahrudak. Perhaps I should have exercised more caution, but I was so close to home and everything seemed unchanged, at least on the surface. Two hours later I found myself on the streets of Navahrudak, on my way to my mother's apartment. I glanced around the square, taking in all the activity and the bustling crowds, and then my heart stopped. There before me was my mother. I flung myself into her arms, and without speaking we started walking. She whispered, "I will take you home, son." We could not express our tangle of emotions with words.

At her two-bedroom apartment I remarked on the sparse furnishings and fittings. She explained that under the current conditions no one was allowed private accommodations, and articles of value were seen as unnecessary trappings. A Soviet nurse now lived with her. After we had given free rein to our joy at being reunited, my mother told me that her roommate was a Communist informant. A grim new vision of Belarus unfolded in my mind as she spoke. Soviet protection had eliminated civil liberties, abolished free speech, and ravaged the lives of successful people. Landowners, teachers, activists, and many politicians had disappeared without a trace. Some had resurfaced in camps in the northern regions of Siberia. A pall of darkness and festering distrust had fallen over my homeland. Soviet authorities had confiscated many goods manufactured in Belarus, weakening the local economy. Agents of the occupying Red Army blindly obeyed their superiors in Moscow. My mother expressed her fear for my safety, instructing me to go to City Hall to register and get the necessary documents. Soviet agents might not accept my explanation about escaping from a German POW camp. Arrest and prosecution was a real danger.

At about nine o'clock that evening the Soviet nurse returned to the apartment. My mother introduced us, and the nurse gave me a faint smile and closeted herself in her bedroom. Now the tone and content of our conversation changed. We talked about family in Lubcza, and I told my mother that my desire to enter medical school had sustained me all these many months. I resolved to go to Lwow, a city in the Soviet Ukraine, where my friends Joe Sazyc and Janka Hutor were studying medicine.

Early the next day I paid a visit to my good friend Janka Pleskacz. We had attended the same gymnasium and shared ideas about preserving our Belarusian culture. Janka believed that I had died on the front, and he was astonished to see me. I blurted out my story and spoke of my plans to enter medical school. He studied me gravely and then told me to sit down. First warning me not to repeat any part of our conversation to anyone, he reiterated what Koscik's uncle and my mother had said about the dramatic changes that had occurred in my absence. Students suspected of anti-Communist sympathies disappeared without a trace, he said, and he was sorry that I had returned. However, he did offer some practical advice about how I could get a passport, which involved speaking to a girl named Abramowicz, a former Jewish classmate from our gymnasium days who worked at City Hall.

When Janka and I parted I headed for City Hall and sought out Abramowicz, who told me that I was to pose as a citizen of another city wishing to register in Navahrudak. Within minutes she presented me with a new passport, which identified me as a full-fledged citizen of Soviet Belarus. I thanked her, and she discreetly suggested that we meet later. We spent a pleasant evening at a local restaurant, carefully avoiding any reference to the prevailing political situation. She told me she was engaged to one of my old school friends. The next time I saw her she was marching with a column of other Jews condemned to death by the German SS.

Before I left for Lwow my mother and I travelled to Lubcza to see family and to visit my father's grave. As I stood beside the grave I contemplated my mother's devotion and the help she so willingly gave me, her family, and anyone who needed it. I was determined not to let her down. A few days later I arrived in Lwow only to discover that I was too late to register for medical school, but Joe Sazyc and Janka Hutor urged me to enter any faculty I could in order to legitimize my presence in the city. They explained that I risked deportation or even death if I returned to Belarus. We had a few short, happy days together, but I decided despite their warnings to return to Navahrudak and take a teaching job in Lubcza. I wanted to work for a year and then apply to medical school the following September.

Back in Lubcza all seemed the same as ever. Settling into my new life there, I was flooded with memories – the river, the forests, the countryside evoked my happy and carefree childhood. Even my grandmother was unchanged. But the robust and domineering grandfather I remembered had entered his own private world. Today I understand that senility likely accounted for his frequent and unprovoked outbursts of anger and irritability.

The beautiful Nabokov Palace, once the home of the Navahrudak gentry, had been converted into a high school, and I heard rumours about the disappearance of the Nabokov family – many people simply assumed that they had ended up in Siberia. (After the war, I learned that the youngest son had managed to get to Germany and make his way to the United States, where he died in 1987.) Miklailow, the high school's Russian director, interviewed me in late September 1940. I apologized for not speaking Russian and foolishly commented that I was surprised that the school had a Russian-language requirement because the majority of its students came from Belarusian backgrounds. Scowling, Miklailow asked me if I was a nationalist who refused to speak Russian. I explained that I was not a nationalist, but I felt very comfortable speaking my own language, especially since the formation of the Belarusian Soviet Socialist Republic. I added that I would willingly learn Russian,

German, Latin, or any other language but emphasized that Belarusians had the right to speak their own language. I worried that I had not made a good impression, but there was a severe shortage of qualified teachers, and the director's superiors demanded that life in the area appear "normal," so he needed me. Despite his suspicions about my nationalist leanings, he grudgingly offered me the low-paying teaching position, and I accepted.

The following the day the director took me aside and asked me if I was the nephew of Bazyl Ragula, who was teaching Russian at this very school. I nodded, and Miklailow retorted that perhaps my uncle was the source of my subversive ideas. I did not reply. I knew that Uncle Bazyl had studied in Russia and spoke the language fluently. He enjoyed Russian literature and poetry, and once, when I asked him why as a Belarusian patriot he valued Russian works, he explained that their words and ideas possessed a singular beauty. After an uneasy silence I assured the director that my uncle had not imparted his political views to me – I had seen little of him when I was growing up. This seemed to mollify the director, but I could not suppress my sense of foreboding.

Under the gymnasium system the high school curriculum spanned a ten-year period. Upon graduation students were expected to possess the necessary skills to enter university. I taught these students, and I also organized their sporting activities – gymnastics, basketball, volleyball, and cross-country skiing. A young Russian teacher, Misha, expressed his support for my work. One day, during a ten-minute break between classes, he invited me to take a walk with him, and as we walked he asked me whether I was enjoying my new teaching position. Then he came to the point: he wanted to warn me that the extra effort I was making to engage the students in sports had planted seeds of suspicion among my superiors. He told me that he was a member of Komsomol, a Communist youth organization, and this was the first step towards becoming a member of the Communist Party. Now, he continued, if I were to join Komsomol too, I would find that I had better opportunities. I mulled this over. Misha was persuasive, but I was afraid. I had heard that candidates for membership in Komsomol were subjected to a thorough investigation. Because I had re-entered Belarus illegally, I feared not only for my own safety but also for that of my loved ones. I smiled at Misha and thanked him. I said that I would give the matter serious thought.

At home that evening I told Aunt Luba about Misha's overtures. She fretted and spoke tearfully about my relationship to my father's brother, Bazyl – a relationship that would pose many problems. Later that evening Uncle Bazyl joined us, and I repeated my story. He stressed that I must not join Komsomol because if I did then I would become inextricably bound up in the heinous Communist political machine. Without hesitation I accepted his advice. I would have to devise a way to keep Misha at arm's length.

Weeks passed in an easy, natural rhythm. I spent many happy, solitary hours in the countryside, I wandered along the Nieman River, and I skied whenever the opportunity presented itself. Then, in early December of 1940, Miklailow called me to his office to discuss my German-language course. We discussed some routine matters related to textbooks and materials, and then Miklailow asked me to explain how I had managed to return to Belarus. My mind raced. I knew that there was no point in denying my escape from Germany, but I had to reveal as few details as possible. I explained that because I was a prisoner of war, I had felt safe in returning to my homeland. When the director asked if I had reported my escape to the authorities, I sidestepped the question and recounted how I had gone to City Hall in Navahrudak to get my papers. There was a strained silence after that, and my heart hammered against my rib cage. Finally Miklailow asked me if I had reached a decision about joining Komsomol. Displaying as much earnestness as I could, I said that I needed more time to study and understand the Communist ideology – unlike the director himself, I was a novice with no political training. With a terse nod he dismissed me, and I left his office convinced that the Communists would now be looking into my activities, both past and present.

When I told my family about this meeting Aunt Luba declared that I must leave immediately for a big city where I might find anonymity. Bristling, I told her that I had committed no crime and that if I disappeared then the Soviets would simply take revenge on my family. So I continued to teach and organize sporting activities, slipping back into my comfortable routine. Shortly before Christmas I visited my cousin Vladimir, Aunt Luba's son, who was six years older than I was. Although Vladimir had aspired to be a veterinarian he had become involved with a bad element, possibly experimenting with drugs and alcohol, and he never completed his education. He had taken a job as a forest ranger, and he lived deep in the woods. I skied to his home, and during my visit I came to appreciate his isolated and undemanding way of life. I also appreciated the male companionship and found myself sharing my past experiences and present concerns with Vladimir.

Christmas in Lubcza that year was a quiet affair, marred only by my mother's continuing fear for my safety. I did all I could to assure her that there was no cause for concern and urged her to enjoy the time we had with Uncle Bazyl, Aunt Luba, Vladimir, and his sister, Nina. When the holidays were over I returned to the gymnasium, where I struck up a friendship with a Soviet teacher. She fell ill, and I brought her delicacies baked by my grandmother. I went to see her one evening after she had recovered, and she placed a bottle of vodka and a dish of herring on the table. Then she announced that we should register as husband and wife. (At the time, one simply had to pay three rubles to the City Hall clerk in order to get married; for thirty rubles, one could just as easily obtain a divorce.) Stammering with surprise, I told her as gently as possible that I could offer her my friendship but nothing more. Unintentionally, I had offended her. Her attitude changed abruptly, and she demanded that I leave and never visit her again. From that night on she refused to acknowledge me when our paths crossed.

Shortly afterwards, on 20 January 1941, Comrade Sokolow, the school supervisor, approached me in the staff dining hall. Although he could see that I had just started my meal, he insisted that he needed to speak with me about my sporting activities. Knowing that it would be unwise to try to put him off, I pulled on my winter coat and the fur hat my mother had given me for Christmas and followed him to Zamkawaja Street. Sokolow politely invited me into a building on the pretext of finding a warm spot to have our conversation. I did not know that this building was the seat of the NKVD operations and that those who entered through its doors usually disappeared.[1]

Sokolow ushered me into a reception area, where he introduced me to the chief of the NKVD – the People's Commissariat of Internal Affairs – who asked me if I would be interested in teaching cross-country skiing to new recruits. I agreed to take on this extra duty during the weekends and afternoons when I did not have to teach. Then the chief instructed Sokolow to wait in the reception area while he and I discussed the details in his office. We proceeded to the office, and as we entered I saw that two armed soldiers were guarding the door. The chief pushed me into a chair, extracted some documents from his pocket, and announced that I was under arrest. The world stood still. Reeling with shock, I asked what I was being accused of, but the chief merely replied that I would be held overnight.

As I sat in a dark, cramped cell, my mind reverberated with the many warnings I had so confidently shrugged off. Faces clouded by terror, panic in the eyes of an old farmer, images of my senile grandfather – oh, how these glimpses of the past tormented me!

During the night guards brought me bread and coffee. Early in the morning my cousin Nina brought food, a change of clothing, and a sweater, but we were forbidden to speak to one another. Then, at about 7:30 a.m., two guards escorted me to the train station. They warned me not to speak to anyone. In a daze, I obeyed, and the three of us boarded a train. I remember arriving in Navahrudak, and then I found myself in prison in Baranovichi. Guards took away my shoelaces, belt, watch, and identification papers and threw me into a cell. Beside me was an excrement-filled pail. As a newcomer to this hellhole, I had been accorded a place of honour.

In the late afternoon I was served a supper of very salty fish and thin barley soup. The salt burned my throat, and I asked the guards for water. They growled at me to keep quiet, that I would get something to drink in due time. Suddenly the cell door swung open and a brusque voice called my name. I was led through corridors by guards whose faces I never saw because they had ordered me to keep my head down. In what appeared to be an interrogation room, I looked about me and saw a desk, a chair, and a Soviet flag. In front of the desk was a high stool. Someone shoved me onto the stool, and the next thing I remember was a NKVD officer standing behind the desk, looking back at me. The guards left quietly.

The officer smiled and asked me if I wanted a cigarette. I croaked out a request for water, but he told me that once we had cleared up a few points, I would get everything I desired. And so began a seemingly endless, soul-devouring relay of interrogations and beatings. Although the inquisitors changed, the questions they fired at me were much the same. What was my name? What did my mother do? How did I get to Lubcza? What was it like being a prisoner of war? How had I crossed the border? As I repeated my answers, carefully avoiding any mention of how I had found a way to breach the heavily guarded border, I became increasingly disoriented. Lack of water, fatigue, and the unrelenting round of questions sent spears of pain though my body. The Communist apes took great pleasure in my discomfort. They grabbed carafes of water and drank, letting the liquid run down their chins and onto their shirt fronts. "Boris," they said, "if you would like some water, all you have to do is sign the confession." Somewhere deep within my spirit I found the strength to resist. I answered each agent in the same way, saying that I could not confess to spying or counter-revolutionary activity because I had not done these things. In defiance, I claimed that I was not thirsty. Then I put my head down and decided to say nothing more.

At each session my interrogators tried different tactics. Some characterized my Uncle Bazyl as a political firebrand, others insisted that my mother wanted me to confess, and as their poisonous words filled the room, I slipped into a state of otherness. I dreamed of fishing, of fighting on the front line, of escaping from the POW camp. Isolated moments from a not-so-distant past whirled through my mind. Had I spoken aloud, or was I plummeting into an abyss of despair – or insanity? Vicious blows to my head brought me back to that vile interrogation room. But still I refused to speak. One NKVD interrogator pulled out his gun, held it to my temple, and told me that my life was worth seven kopeks. I heard the trigger click, and I sat mute and motionless on the stool. Yet another officer came into the room. What transpired next is a blur. I awoke in a cell with thirty or forty other prisoners, and the sickening stench from a pail of excrement assaulted my senses.

Next to me sat a man of about sixty-five. His blue eyes were kind and he had a pleasant expression. He asked me my name and called me Boris Dimitrievich, a term of endearment. He gave me water and bread, watched me consume this meagre repast, and then gently massaged my forehead and back. When he asked me why I was in prison I told him about crossing the border and meeting the crazed farmer who had warned me to return to the Germans. It was as if I had finally pushed against the weak point in some internal dam – all of my hatred for the Soviet occupiers spilled out. The man cradled me in his arms for some time, and then he told me that I would pay a very high price for my ideas. He said he was sorry for me. I craved human comfort and a release from the interminable torture of my interrogators, so I opened up to this man. I had no inkling of his evil purpose.

Years later I learned that while the NKVD detained me at their headquarters four uniformed agents had descended upon my grandparents' home. They threatened every member of the household and systematically ransacked the small dwelling, ostensibly looking for weapons and evidence of anti-Communist activity. They destroyed furniture, pillows, books, letters, and even the contents of the larder. Unable to comprehend this violation of her home, my grandmother knelt in prayer. One agent called her a stupid old woman and told her that God could not help her because her grandson was an enemy of the Soviet state. When the agents had left my family silently set about putting the house in order. After a few hours, when most of the evidence of the intrusion had been cleared away, Aunt Luba suggested that they contact my mother.

They managed to get a call through to her at the hospital the next day. My mother, wasting little time, changed into her civilian clothes and rushed to the local police station. She gave the officer on duty information about my arrest in Lubcza and demanded to know where the authorities had taken me. When the officer denied all knowledge of the incident she became even more aggressive and insistent. Finally he ordered her to leave at once or face interrogation for her activities in Hramada, a social democratic youth organization that supported Belarusian arts and culture. My mother refused to back down, and the officer literally tossed her out of the police station.

She boarded a train for Lubcza and went straight to NKVD headquarters, where she presented herself to the officer on duty. He confirmed my arrest. When she insisted on an explanation, he told her to leave. With no other recourse, she went to her parents' house. Later, family members told me that it was the first time they had ever seen my mother sobbing.

While my family struggled to cope with their uncertainty and terror, I languished in a prison cell. One evening a guard opened my cell door and told me to put on my coat. Then he thrust my hands in irons. In the dark courtyard I saw the outline of a truck with prisoners sitting in the back. A soldier pushed me into the crowded vehicle. We arrived, some hours later, in Minsk, the capital of the Belarusian Soviet Socialist Republic. We were herded into a prison and subjected to a body search. An officer explained that the accusations against me included collaborating with the Belarusian nationalist bourgeoisie, entering the Soviet Union illegally, engaging in anti-Communist activity, spying for the Germans, hiding arms, and inciting an armed uprising against the Soviet Union. I was instructed to sign a document attesting to the fact that I had read the charges, but I refused, declaring that the accusations were lies. I was told to shut up and prepare myself to be interrogated; once the investigators had reviewed my case, I would be informed of the result. Lacking the strength to resist I shuffled along prison corridors and up a winding staircase. I was shoved into a cell – I still remember that it was number 17 – and the door slammed shut behind me. I was alone.

I peered at my surroundings. A strong lamp stood next to a folding bed. In one corner a table was affixed to the wall. I smiled wryly when I spotted a pail, but this one was empty. A guard slid open a latch door and shouted at me to go to sleep. I pulled down the folding bed, flopped onto the straw mattress, and dozed off quickly, but soon I was writhing with discomfort. Bed bugs were crawling all over me. I rolled on the floor, trying to rid myself of this infestation, but the same guard heard me and ordered me back to bed. In the morning I complained about the bugs, and to my surprise I was given an instrument with which to burn them, and eventually I received a new mattress. Daily rations consisted of water and some wet, sticky bread. My spirits crumbled. My dreams, my family, my life receded. Perhaps my NKVD tormentors had been right and my life was of little worth.

Several nights later a guard escorted me to a windowless room furnished with a desk and a high stool. A smartly dressed officer entered the room and spoke pleasantly about how I could begin a new life if I showed remorse for my crimes. I told him what I had told the other interrogators, and then there was nothing more to say. Ignoring my silence, the officer asked me what I knew of Belarusian history. Unaware of the trap, I started to talk about the Grand Duchy of Lithuania and the Belarusian Rada. There was an eerie silence, and then my interrogator remarked that I had obviously been brainwashed. Everything I had told him about Belarus led him to believe that I was an agent for revolutionary groups bent on the destruction of the Soviet state.

Weeks passed, each day blurring into the next. Depression enveloped me. I made a chess set out of bread and tried to play my left hand against my right. Mental diversion suddenly seemed vital, as did physical activity. I ran on the spot and did push-ups and callisthenics. I started to lose weight. One night, possibly during February 1941, guards led me to an interrogation room in the basement of the prison – again outfitted with desk and stool. A burly NKVD officer entered, and I quavered at the sight of him. Solid build, dark hair, curved nose, pointed chin, cruel lips – the man inspired revulsion. Without looking at me, he flicked through a file and told me that his name was Isaac Ginsberg. Suddenly he sprang towards me, yelling that I had lied. He thrust the papers into my hand and demanded that I read them. As I started to read my heart sank. My compassionate older cellmate in the Baranovichi prison had provided a detailed account of our conversation. Other entries in the file were pure fiction. It took me about half an hour to read the notes; I closed the folder and told Ginsberg that the author was a liar. He took great pleasure in beating me. Gasping for breath, reeling from his powerful blows, I found myself once again on the stool. Again Ginsberg repeated the charges against me, and again I refused to sign a confession. Blackness swallowed me. When I regained my senses my interrogator had gone. Two guards dragged me to another cell in the bowels of the prison. Ginsberg's fists and boots had inflicted damage on practically every part of my body. Moisture glistened on the stone walls of the cell. This was isolation. Some days later a guard came to take me back to my old cell.

I was left undisturbed for several days, and then I was hauled back to the now-familiar interrogation room. A smiling young lieutenant entered, and in a friendly tone he told me that I had had an unfortunate misunderstanding with my last interrogator. He hoped that I had now learned to control my emotions. He encouraged me, as a friend, to sign the confession. I raised my head and looked into his eyes. I trusted no one. When I shook my head in refusal he spewed a litany of Soviet propaganda. He told me that the Soviets would eliminate people like me who wanted to destroy the state from within.

The round of interrogations continued. At times I would be left alone in my cell for two or three days, and then I would be returned to the interrogation room. One night – by my reckoning it was at the end of March 1941 – I was taken to a different room, one equipped with a bench and leather straps. Two low-ranking NKVD men and the loathsome Ginsberg were there waiting for me. Ginsberg glared menacingly at me, and then he passed me the file saying I had one last chance to reconsider. If I did not confess, then I would have to face the consequences of my actions. I told him again that I had nothing to confess. The two NKVD lackeys grabbed me and strapped me face down to the bench. They removed my shoes. A drilling pain shot through my legs and dulled my senses, and finally I fell into darkness. When I came to, water was dripping from my head and I was sitting on the bench. Ginsberg ordered me to stand, but when I tried to do so I fell to the floor. He barked at me to put my shoes on, and I saw that my feet were terribly swollen. Before the guards dragged me back to my cell, Ginsberg leered into my face and spit out a warning that this was just a taste of things to come. Slowly my feet healed, but Ginsberg's torture had emptied my soul. I feared that I would one day succumb to the NKVD in order to end my physical and emotional torment.

For some reason I was allowed books. Most of the materials supplied to prisoners exalted Communist ideals, so I left them on the librarian's cart. I did, however, find several books of verse, which I studied carefully. I memorized lengthy verses, knowing that I needed some kind of intellectual diversion in order to survive. In May the round of futile interrogations resumed. On one occasion the hateful Ginsberg stated in a deathly calm voice that for people like me there was nothing left but death. He took out a gun and said that guards would take me to an isolated place not far from Minsk and end my life with a single bullet.[2] I knew now that I would either be executed or deported. A few days later I was delivered to a room in which three NKVD officers sat behind a long desk. One began to read from a document listing my crimes, ending his lengthy recitation with the words, "You are condemned to death by firing squad." Another officer asked me if I had anything to say. Numbly, I shook my head. He pushed a document towards me and told me to sign it. I asked him if this meant that I was confessing. He replied that the document simply confirmed that I was aware of the charges against me. I signed. Then the officer informed me that I had thirty days to appeal to Stalin for clemency, and that my death sentence could be commuted to twenty-five years in a labour camp. I clung to this slight ray of hope – a lot could happen in thirty days.

That night I joined nine other prisoners on death row. There was writing etched into the concrete cell wall. Our predecessors had left a record of their names and dates and the charges that had landed them in this desolate place.

On the morning of 22 June 1941 we heard explosions. Someone suggested that it was a military exercise, but I thought differently. With each blast, the walls shook. A lad of eighteen or so joined us in the cell. He cried out with excitement, "Comrades! The Germans are bombing Minsk!" Some of us feared that the NKVD would begin slaughtering all prisoners, but on the second day of bombing guards led us into the prison yard and then into the city streets. Everywhere I looked I saw ruined and burning buildings. I also spotted another group of prisoners, perhaps 10,000 in number, and as the bombs fell I moved towards them. Someone called for all the American prisoners to come forward, so I kept my head down and followed the Americans. The guards pointed us eastward, in the direction of Czerwien, about sixty kilometres from Minsk.

Any prisoner who fell behind was shot and killed. I was thankful that I had managed to stay in relatively good physical condition. We arrived at the Czerwien prison, and there a commissar for the NKVD announced that each of us would be checked by name and by type of crime committed. Having witnessed the disarray of the Soviet Army in Minsk, I did not believe that the NKVD had the necessary files and documents to do this. I watched and listened as the tallying and checking process proceeded. Three NKVD agents sat at a table with blank sheets of paper before them. As each prisoner came forward an agent would write down his name and place him in one of two crime categories: espionage or anti-Communist activity; or domestic crimes of a minor nature. Those in the first group were heavily guarded and ordered to stand by a stone wall. Stepping up to the table, I invented a name for myself. When asked what my crime was, I said that I did not know, but that I had been ordered to work in the woods and produce a quota of cordwood; due to a chest infection, I had not been able to do the work and was sent to prison. I spoke in simple, peasant language and pretended to be stupid. The agent ordered me to join the larger, less closely guarded group of prisoners. I obediently took my place among them and sat down to rest my tired body. By the end of the day we had seen some 1,100 prisoners lined up against the wall, and by late evening they had all disappeared. I heard the staccato blare of machine-gun fire and assumed that it was a military engagement with the invading Germans, but I was later told by local peasants that what I had heard was a mass execution: the NKVD had shot the 1,100 prisoners in an area east of Czerwien.

At about 4 a.m. we heard someone shout that the guards had disappeared. We all rose to our feet in an uproarious clamour and threw open the prison gates. Then I ran. I ran until I could run no further, and then I crept into the root cellar of an isolated farmhouse. I remained there one day and one night. When at last I emerged from my hideaway, I was amazed to see a German tank with a four-man crew in the farmyard. The men were shaving. Apprehensively, I approached them and bid them good morning in German. They asked me who I was, and I explained that I had been released from a Soviet prison and wanted to return to my family in a village west of Minsk. Since I spoke German, they said, I could be on my way – I needed no special travel documents.

I journeyed west, and no one stopped me or even spoke to me. I saw unarmed Soviet soldiers in retreat, and there was little evidence of military discipline or order in their frantic escape from the Germans. On my approach to Minsk, I saw two German soldiers at the crossroads standing at ease, guns by their sides, beside a massive pile of Soviet weapons. They were accepting the surrender of Soviet soldiers and letting them go. At another site I saw a troop of German soldiers executing prisoners of war. West of Minsk I saw villagers coming out of their homes with bread and salt on white towels, greeting the German soldiers and hailing them as liberators. Others had lit candles before their treasured icons and were offering prayers of thanks to God for bringing Stalin's cruel reign to an end. The world no longer made sense to me. I continued to walk.

3 Liberation?

On my long journey home I had little difficulty finding food and lodging. When people learned that I had escaped from a Soviet prison, they generously opened their homes to me, and many called me a hero. Almost every family I met along the way told me stories of how the Soviets had massacred civilians, deported people, and confiscated property, all in the name of Communism, but thoughts of my own family, especially my mother, remained uppermost in my mind.

Finally I reached the outskirts of the town of Naliboki, part of the Polish territory. Local police, who were under German command, had orders to infiltrate all organizations in order to preserve and advance the Polish cause. When a police officer stopped me and asked me where I had come from, I gave few details but said that I had been in a Soviet prison. Hesitantly, I added that I would give further information to his commander. Once again, threatened and unsure of my fate, I found myself in a guarded room in a police station. An attendant brought me to meet the unit's commanding officer. I was thunderstruck – there behind the desk was Eugene Klimowicz, another friend from the gymnasium. In an even voice, he asked me who I was, and it dawned on me that few people would recognize the gaunt, dirty, and bewhiskered shadow of a man I had become. Prison life had ravaged my body. I addressed him quietly by name and reminded him of my cousin Nina, my aunt Luba, the summers we had spent swimming and fishing together in Lubcza. Recognition flooded through him, and we embraced as old friends.

Eugene explained that as commanding officer of this unit, his intention was to eradicate the Communists and, if possible, punish them for their crimes. I told him about the shattered Red Army forces retreating in droves and lurking in wooded areas. He gave me a friendly shake and said that this was no time to talk politics. I was alive, and we were reunited. When he offered me a drink, I declined. Seeing how exhausted I was, he arranged for me to have what I sorely needed – a bath, clean clothes, good food, and a warm bed. I slept soundly that night.

Early the next morning Eugene and I had breakfast together, and as we ate I asked if he had any news of my family. When he told me that he had lost touch due to the upheaval of war, I suspected that he was being evasive because Lubcza was only twenty-five kilometres away. Later that day he hired a farmer with a horse and wagon to take me home, but after about five kilometres, the farmer ordered me out of the wagon. I resisted, and he swore at me, saying that he would not risk travelling through forested areas because the NKVD and the Soviets might still be hiding in the area. He raised his horsewhip, so I jumped off the wagon and continued on foot.

As I walked through this lovely natural area, I felt renewed in spirit and soul. I lingered on the riverbanks, listened to the songbirds, and recalled the sun-filled days I had passed here with friends and relatives. Tears streaming down my face, I climbed over my grandfather's fence, walked past the vegetable garden and the orchard, and approached the door to my home, where I stood paralyzed by emotion. Suddenly Aunt Luba threw open the door, and when she found her voice she called out to my grandparents. Embracing them, I was filled with overpowering feelings of love, loss, and relief. They had so many questions for me, but I had only one for them: "Where is my mother?" A despairing silence filled the room. Finally Aunt Luba explained that my mother had died when German bombs hit the hospital in Navahrudak. She had been evacuating patients. She had died fulfilling her duty to her patients, just as my father had done so many years earlier. Sobs racked my whole being.

Eventually I found the strength to ask Aunt Luba where my mother was buried, and she told me that her sister lay in the military cemetery at Navahrudak. I announced that I would bring her home to rest beside my father and my brother. I have little recollection of what occurred that evening, but I know that Aunt Luba drew me a bath and cried when she saw the scars on my back. She said nothing, but she dried my back and covered it with healing kisses. Such a simple act of love gave purpose to my life.

After resting for a week, I set out to bring my mother's body back to Lubcza. On the journey, my memories, my dreams, and the promises I had made to my mother tumbled together in my anguished mind. I was overcome by a sense of helplessness and sorrow. At Navahrudak I sought out a nurse who had worked with my mother, and she described the German attack for me. At about ten o'clock on the morning of 22 June 1941, wave after wave of German Stuka bombers appeared from the west. They destroyed almost 75 per cent of the city. With the roads blocked by the fleeing Soviet administrators and NKVD ranks, confusion, panic, and chaos spread rapidly through the civilian population. My mother helped some patients out of the hospital and into a nearby park, then she turned back to help others. Debris from a bomb ripped into her skull. She fell, holding a patient, who miraculously survived. Knowing the circumstances of my dear mother's death gave me no solace.

At the Belarusian City Hall, I obtained the necessary permit. Although I had no money, I offered some city employees compensation for helping me transport my mother's body to Lubcza. Silently, I watched them dig up the body, which was wrapped only in a hospital sheet. We placed her gently in a coffin, loaded it onto a wagon, and slowly undertook the six-hour walk to Lubcza. When we arrived my grandmother insisted on calling the priest to say some prayers. I did not care – for me, prayers had no healing power, but perhaps they would comfort my grandmother and Aunt Luba. We took my mother to the cemetery and laid her beside her beloved husband. At last they were both at peace.

One day passed into the next. Nothing interested me. We learned that my Uncle Czetyrko had been deported and that Uncle Bazyl had managed to escape from a Soviet prison. Most of the Belarusian intelligentsia had been rounded up, loaded onto cattle cars, and deported east. I avoided thinking or speaking about the political situation. I felt dull and depleted. I met Natasha, a former girlfriend, and we took walks and bike rides together. One day she told me that she was married. I was shocked. During the Soviet occupation, when people were suffering from a lack of food and other necessities of life, Natasha had married an influential man who worked in the city administration. Although she admitted that she did not love him, she felt compelled to marry him because he was in charge of food distribution. Survival, not sentiment, had governed her choice, and I was in no position to judge her. However, when she told me that she wanted to have my child, I severed ties with her. I could not in good conscience take advantage of her unhappiness.

My cousin Michael, Uncle Bazyl's son, came from Lwow, where he was studying engineering, and he told me about the nationalist revival in Ukraine. Ukrainian nationals had declared independence, but the Germans had revoked it. Nonetheless, the Ukrainians were striving to rebuild their schools and create a local constabulary and armed forces under German supervision. Michael believed strongly that the time had come for Belarusians to re-establish their national identity and revive the cultural and social institutions that had been suppressed during the Soviet occupation. I listened to him listlessly, but gradually his youthful optimism and patriotic fire stirred my own nationalist fervour. I asked Uncle Bazyl what he thought about the future of Belarus. When he had held seats in the Polish Parliament and Senate, he had co-operated with the German minority, which at the time had supported democratic principles. He responded to my question by saying that the Germans would restructure the Soviet Union in such a way as to allow Belarus to prosper as an independent and self-governing nation. Shortly after that he spoke at a meeting in Lubcza's town square, which I attended. He emphasized the strength of Belarus and then stepped down from the wagon that served as a speaking platform saying that I, his nephew, had an important message for the audience – a crowd of Belarusian farmers. I was totally unprepared to address the assembly. In fact, I had never spoken in public before. But once I began to express my disgust for the Soviet regime, all my inhibitions dissipated. My words drew enthusiastic applause. Somehow I felt reborn, and my long-dormant passion for political activism rose within me.

There followed a time of waiting and watching as the Germans moved eastward. By the end of September 1941, Hitler's armies had reached Smolensk, a city on the eastern border of Belarus. General Brauchnitz, commander of the German ground forces, suggested that the eastward march be halted to allow the Germans to organize a buffer zone consisting of Ukraine, Belarus, and the Baltic nations. Brauchnitz understood the need to establish regional depots where local produce and other supplies could be channelled through to the eastern front, but the high command in Berlin removed him from the front, despite the strong support his plan received from high-ranking officers in the Ostministerium (the Ministry for the Occupied East). Apparently Hitler intended to have tea in Moscow by the end of November.

When I discussed these occurrences with Uncle Bazyl in September 1941, he postulated that Hitler was committing the same mistake that had led to Napoleon's 1812 defeat. He also predicted that the Germans' failure would be a pivotal event in the course of the war. Other politically aware people shared his views. I visited a colleague of my uncle's named Godlewski, and we discussed the implications of Germany's aggressive movement on the eastern front. Godlewski, a priest, expressed his wariness of the German Reich. Based on what he had seen in other occupied territories, he believed that Belarus would have some limited freedoms under the Germans, but there would also be jurisdictional conflicts. Nonetheless, he held fast to his hope that Belarus would one day achieve independence.

Because I had escaped from a Soviet prison and spoke fluent German, the mayor of Navahrudak welcomed me with open arms. He wanted me to act as interpreter and liaison between Belarusian citizens and the newly formed German administration. When I agreed, he introduced me to Stabsleiter Wolfmyer, a short, stocky man wearing a brown uniform and a swastika arm band. Although Wolfmyer professed a willingness to establish German authority with benevolence, not violence, I remained guarded in my actions and words – for one thing, I did not mention to him that I had been a prisoner of war in Germany – yet somehow Wolfmyer and I developed an easy working relationship. In preparation for the arrival of the German commissar for the area, he and I made several trips to Vilnius to buy furnishings and other goods. Wolfmyer also found me very useful to have around because I could converse in Polish and Russian, as well as German and Belarusian. When I voiced my concern for the plight of Belarusians who were being persecuted by Polish administrators and wrongfully charged with being pro-

Communist, Wolfmyer took it upon himself to investigate, and he promised to notify me of any charges against citizens suspected of Communist activity. He reasoned that since I was well known in the area, I would be able to determine the validity of such charges.

When my good friend Joe Sazyc returned from Lwow, I tried to convince him to take the job of commander of the Navahrudak police because he would provide a Belarusian presence. He firmly refused, stating that after what he had seen in Ukraine he did not believe that the Germans would sanction independent status for Belarus. German occupying forces had rounded up Ukrainian nationalists and sent them to concentration camps. Joe's account disturbed me deeply. It now seemed likely to me that the Germans intended to exploit Belarus as a link in their much needed eastern supply line, but our choices were severely limited – we Belarusians could not go back to the Soviets, and we did not have the strength to eject the Germans. And so we waited.

Although achieving primary goals for Belarusian independence seemed next to impossible given the unsettled political situation, a number of townspeople found ways to circumvent the German authorities. A group that included some local teachers organized the Narodny Dom, a community centre where choirs, dance groups, and theatre groups met and where lectures were presented. With the support of Dr Orser, the townspeople proposed to expand the school system to include a gymnasium. When the occupying authorities rejected this plan, the group sent a memorandum to administrators in Navahrudak requesting permission to open a "teachers' college." They won approval for this, and then used the approved teachers' college facilities to quietly implement the Belarusian gymnasium curriculum. Dr Orser was appointed chairman of education in Navahrudak and the surrounding area, and he and his wife worked diligently to lay the groundwork for a well-rounded education system. He organized teachers, created a school-inspection system, and visited every school in the district. He also acted as an ambassador and spokesperson for Belarusian culture. I consider it a privilege to have worked with this man. Dr Orser was my mentor and a true friend.

During conversations with Joe Sazyc, I outlined a plan for providing military training to students enrolled at the gymnasium – or teachers' college, as it was officially called – originally built by Belarusians. The training course would fall under the category of physical education. Many Belarusians still believed that the Germans would require their military assistance to invade Moscow. Joe threw himself into the project with enthusiasm, and soon Belarusian youths were sporting homemade uniforms, practising drills and field manoeuvres, and learning basic elements of planning and strategy. Enrolment exceeded expectations. The school also offered a diverse curriculum, which included math, physics, and Latin and Belarusian language, literature, and history. Although the German authorities had closed all universities in the territory, our core group of teachers and planners understood the importance of giving students every opportunity for a better future.

My friend Janka Hutor had a younger sister named Ludmila who wanted to work to help her family. I knew that the Germans in Navahrudak needed telephone operators, so I told Janka to bring his sister to see me. I remembered Ludmila as a youngster of five or six years old whom Janka and I had teased mercilessly, but when Janka brought her to my office I was moonstruck. Gone was the gawky child, and before me stood a lovely young girl on the threshold of womanhood, with glossy brown hair, a high forehead, sparkling hazel eyes – she was breathtaking. Janka prodded me in the ribs and asked me what I thought. Distracted, I said, "She is gorgeous!" Grimacing, Janka retorted, "You dolt – I meant can you get her a job!" I expedited the paperwork and had Wolfmyer's approval before the end of the day.

In November Ludmila left the job I found for her and enrolled in the teachers' college. She had musical talent as well as an aptitude for the arts. Since she was only sixteen, I promised her father that I would look after her while she studied in Navahrudak. The Hutors had a home in Navahrudak, but Mr Hutor was a school inspector, which meant that he often had to travel to outlying towns and villages. With Dr Orser's help, we found Ludmila an apartment in the block that I lived in. I knew that I would have to bide my time, but I promised myself that when she was older, and if she loved me as I loved her, Ludmila would be my wife.

After routing the Red Army, the Germans converted the collective farms into small land holdings. In theory, farmers who operated these small enterprises would sell a percentage of their produce to the German armed forces. In practice, the Germans confiscated the produce and left the farmers barely enough to survive on. Many POWs from the Soviet Union fled to the buffer zones in Belarus and Ukraine, where they easily found work as farm labourers. Gradually, the German command came to suspect these itinerants of organizing a Communist resistance. Rather than face the deprivation and possible death that awaited them in POW camps, many of these desperate prisoners – known as "partisan guerrillas" – went into hiding. Initially they had no ideological motivation, they were merely bent on survival, but later some of them inflicted hardship upon local inhabitants, inspiring fear in them. However, other members of the guerrilla bands refused to use violence against innocent civilians.

An itinerant POW called Victor, who later joined the guerrillas, found work on the Hutor family farm. Mrs Hutor had remained in the country to run the farm with Victor's help while her husband worked in the educational system. Family members in the town relied on the farm produce because there were serious shortages of food. Eventually Victor decided to leave the farm and join the guerrillas because he was afraid that he would be imprisoned by the Germans, but before he left he promised Mrs Hutor that he would do everything in his power to keep her and her family safe.

Word reached us that Victor's guerrilla band, unlike other notorious bands, never executed farmers or abused village women; he and his cohorts presented themselves as a regular army unit and abided by the highest military standards.

I continued to teach German and military arts at the gymnasium. Wolfmyer kept his promise, and I was permitted to interview anyone suspected of pro-Communist activities. I discovered that many of the accused were guilty only of unbridled patriotism, not Communism. I also worked as the interpreter for Commissar Traub, whose main duty was to develop a reliable and efficient supply of goods for the German army on the eastern front. On many occasions I tried to persuade Traub to support the revival of Belarusian political and social autonomy, and he would express his sympathy and explain that he had no power to change Germany's eastern politics.

In April 1942 Commissar Traub asked me to travel to Germany with him, his wife, and several aides, and I interpreted it as a sign of his trust in me. As we travelled westward by car, I was haunted by memories of my time as a prisoner of war. We stopped at Konigsberg, and I asked Traub if I could take the car and go for a short drive through the countryside. He agreed readily, and I drove straight to the village of Weisendorf, to the farm where I had worked as a POW. I wanted to see Helga again. There was nobody working in the fields when I got there, so, straightening my shoulders, I knocked on the farmhouse door. Helga – the same lovely Helga – answered, and she stood staring at me. She asked if I was Boris. I told her what had happened to me and how I had gained my freedom. As she stepped aside to invite me in, I saw a cradle in the room behind her. She told me that her husband was on the eastern front. I had mixed emotions, but she said that she had only the fondest memories of me, and then I knew she had not betrayed me. I forced myself to leave quickly – she still had the power to tempt me with her charm and her loveliness.

We continued our trip to West Germany, and the commissar granted me unlimited freedom to explore the cities at which we stopped to rest. As I walked through the streets I saw that Jews wore a yellow Star of David and Eastern Europeans wore a yellow badge that read "OST." Soon I learned that these designations identified both groups as undesirable elements in German society. My explorations took me many places, but I particularly sought out POWs who had "volunteered" to work for Germany. Many had come to Germany believing that here they would be given educational opportunities or technical training. One day I stopped a young fellow on the street and asked him who he was and where he was from. He spoke to me in Russian and said that he was one of the foolish ones who had been duped by German promises. He showed me huge, overcrowded barracks where others like him slept on straw mattresses. These people were undernourished, overworked, and downtrodden. Most worked twelve- or fourteen-hour days in labour camps, in ammunition factories, or on railways, and each one I spoke to told me he wanted to go home but feared punishment at the hands of the Germans. At each barracks I visited I heard the same story of misery and oppression, and I began to understand that the Germans considered Jews and Eastern Europeans as sources of forced labour and pawns in the terror apparatus of the regime. Moreover, they had managed to suppress news of all this, leaving Belarusians and other Slavic peoples in ignorance of the events taking place beyond their borders. I vowed to do everything I could to bring an end to the exodus of "volunteers" from Belarus.[1]

Full realization of the goals and ideological foundations of the German Reich came to me when I bought a copy of Hitler's diatribe *Mein Kampf*. Now I understood why the book was unavailable in occupied countries. It shocked me to learn that Hitler intended to conquer the Slavic peoples and enslave them in the service of the superior Aryan race. On the return trip to Navahrudak I struggled with the precarious situation of my homeland. Could we cooperate with the Germans without falling victim to their venomous ambitions? Back in Navahrudak, I set about informing the townspeople of the real situation in Germany. I told a group of young boys at a meeting held in the gymnasium about the forced labour camps and the conditions that I had witnessed, and I explained the ideas expressed in *Mein Kampf*. They understood our predicament right away: we Belarusians could neither back the Communists nor establish a full alliance with the Germans. All we could do was spread the word about what was happening in Germany. Should the German administration force anyone to "volunteer," then we would band together to help this person, even if it meant orchestrating an escape.

News of my dissenting views reached the commissar, and in May 1942 he dismissed me from my post as interpreter. This meant the loss of special privileges such as extra food and liquor rations. Despite my ostracism from the official German administration, Wolfmyer and I remained on good terms. He had fallen in love with a young girl who played an active role in the Belarusian community. Whether it was out of love for her or because he fundamentally disagreed with the German policies, Wolfmyer began warning our loosely organized resistance group about German initiatives to suppress our activities. Unfortunately, even Wolfmyer could not save one of our most active and popular patriots, Panko, the first mayor of Navahrudak. Panko had a weakness for alcohol, and when he drank he often voiced his loathing of the German occupying forces. One day he disappeared. After exhausting every other available method of locating Panko, I asked for a meeting with Commissar Traub. I found my former employer hostile, dismissive, and uninterested in helping me find my friend. I knew then that Panko had been killed.

After Panko's disappearance many of my friends and colleagues realized that our local network of patriots lacked the resources to sustain an effective resistance to the occupying forces. Towards the end of May 1942 I received a call from my friend Vowa, who asked me to come to Minsk for a clandestine meeting, which would take place in early June at the apartment of the local police chief, a man named Sakowiczy. Also attending the meeting were my cousin Michael Ragula; Adamowicz, a literary critic from Minsk; and Szkielonak, another gifted journalist. We took special precautions, arriving at different times, knowing full well that if our purpose were discovered then we would all be sent to the gallows. Out of our heated discussion at that meeting came the underground Belarusian Independence Party (BNP). Through this organization we resolved to develop a network of Belarusian patriots who would try to influence German policies as they applied to conditions in our homeland. Our primary goal was to establish a Belarusian Democratic Republic. We published a journal, the *BNP Bulletin*, the first issue of which appeared in August 1942. I was closely involved in this widely distributed bulletin, and Ludmila helped me to print it and to conceal our illegal activities. In the *BNP Bulletin*, Belarusians first read about the oppressive conditions imposed on "volunteer" workers in Germany as well as Hitler's ideology of eliminating "inferior" races, the extermination of Jews, and Nazi atrocities.

Sakowiczy resigned as police chief of Minsk, and soon afterwards the executive committee of the BNP sent him to Lida, which was the centre of Polish underground activity, to organize the Belarusian national resistance forces. He contacted members of the Polish resistance and convinced them that the Polish and Belarusian undergrounds should join forces against a common enemy – the Soviet Union. While in Poland Sakowiczy also discovered that a few small Polish resistance groups were cooperating with the Germans in return for supplies and ammunition; this cooperation involved fighting the Red Guerrillas, who were causing headaches for the Germans. Attacks by the Red Guerrillas had intensified dramatically, and the German railway police needed both military and locally sanctioned resistance units to protect the flow of goods to the eastern front.

Another member of the BNP, Genko, a graduate of the University of Vilnius, helped to establish the Belarusian Youth Organization. This organization, similar in many respects to the Boy Scout movement, attracted thousands of young people between the ages of thirteen and sixteen. Outwardly, the Belarusian Youth Organization resembled the Soviet and German youth groups whose members wore green uniforms with white-red-white striped arm bands.[2] Soon, Minsk, Vilnius, Navahrudak, Baranovichi, and other towns and villages boasted chapters of the youth group. As coordinator for the organization, Genko travelled extensively, always careful to hide his allegiance to the BNP. He observed conditions in many parts of Belarus and regularly contributed analytical essays to the bulletin about the future of Belarusian culture and self-determination. Despite the escalating threat of the Red Guerrillas, 1941–42 was a golden year for our national aspirations.

4 The Eskadron

By the early autumn of 1943 the Germans knew that they needed the support of the local population to deal with the escalating attacks of the Red Guerrillas. Commissar Traub called the mayors of Lubcza, Dyatlovo, Kareliczy, and Navahrudak to a meeting to "discuss the political situation." All those assembled in the German administration building in Navahrudak looked uncomfortable. When no one responded to his request for suggestions, Traub found himself in the awkward position of consulting my uncle Bazyl. Rather than show false deference to the occupying authorities, my uncle admonished Traub for not asking such questions in 1941. Now that the Red Guerrillas had strengthened their forces with devastating results, it was too late to ask for "suggestions."

Unperturbed by the commissar's glower, Uncle Bazyl reminded him and all present that a solution had been proposed and summarily ignored. Perhaps, he continued, the Germans would like to review the proposal for creating a Belarusian state. Such a political solution would have the advantage of channelling the powerful anti-Communist feeling among the citizens, and it would prompt them to give their wholehearted support for an armed resistance to the Soviets. An uneasy hush descended. Choosing his words carefully, the interpreter translated for the commissar. Traub's expression softened and he slumped forward a little in his chair. It seemed to me at the time that this meeting accomplished very little in the way of defending our civilian population, because the commissar did not pursue my uncle's proposed solution. Upon reflection, however, I believe that Traub hesitated to act because he desperately wanted to believe in the Reich's superiority. To work with Belarusian leaders as equals would be to admit that the German foothold in the territory was unstable.

Not long after that Commissar Traub sent me a message saying that I was to come to see him the next day. I was fearful and suspicious. Were the Germans planning to search my apartment? If they did, then they would find the *BNP Bulletin* and the weapons I had cached there. Ludmila and I quickly hid the incriminating materials, and later that evening I sought advice from Dr Orser, who pointed out that if the Germans did in fact suspect me of illegal activity, then they would have dispensed with the formal invitation – they would have eliminated me, as they had so many others. Although this made sense, I could not conceal my agitation. Dr Orser advised me to meet with Traub, and once we knew what Traub intended, then the two of us would discuss the situation. I slept fitfully that night.

The next morning, dressed in civilian clothes, I set out for Traub's office. To my surprise, his aides redirected me to the commissar's residence. At the entrance to the Traub house, a guard saluted me. The commissar's wife, a very attractive and pleasant woman, greeted me and ushered me into the living room. Soon the commissar joined us and graciously served me a glass of schnapps. He settled into a leather armchair, and we exchanged a few pleasantries. Then Traub explained that he wanted to speak plainly, but he also wanted to apologize for our past misunderstandings. Now, he admitted, he had a better sense of what I had been attempting to communicate since the beginning of his administration. While some within the Reich continued to misunderstand the situation, he believed that under the prevailing conditions the aspirations and national goals of Belarusians were compatible with the goals of the German people. By collaborating, Belarus and Germany could work towards the creation of a new order in the Soviet Union.

We sat in silent contemplation for a few moments. Traub's remarks had taken me completely by surprise. For the first time, the Germans were confessing that they had made strategic errors in their dealings with Belarus. Traub went on to explain that the newly appointed governor general of Belarus, von Gottberg, was seeking the active participation of Belarusians in determining their own future, in defending against the Red Guerrilla threat, and in confronting the approaching danger of the Red Army. To this end, von Gottberg proposed the creation of an independent cavalry unit, stationed in Navahrudak, which would be under my command. Furthermore, continued Traub, I would deal directly with Minsk – remaining independent of the gendarmes and local authorities – and thereby have a free hand in implementing defensive measures to protect Navahrudak from the Red Guerrillas. As much as this proposal pleased me, I tried to remain detached, and I asked for more details. Traub proceeded to outline the basic plan, which called for a cavalry unit of at least 150 men, equipped with modern arms and, more importantly, with unfettered authority to carry out defensive measures under my command. Although I tried to hide my enthusiasm, I could not quell my feelings of triumph. Our civilian population desperately needed protection not only from the Red Guerrillas but also from the German administration. Many of the most dedicated members of the Belarusian intelligentsia had already been deported or exterminated for their nationalist views.

With great self-control, I told Traub that I wanted twenty-four hours to consider the proposal and decide whether I could muster the required manpower.

In the privacy of my apartment, I sat and thought carefully about Traub's proposition. I had no time to call a meeting with my BNP colleagues in Minsk, so I decided that I at least had to consult with Dr Orser, but before I even left for his home I knew that I was already committed to forming what would be called the Eskadron ("cavalry unit" in Belarusian). My good friend Orser welcomed me with open arms. As I laid out Traub's proposal for him, he listened with intense concentration. Although he saw the many benefits that could flow from such a venture, he also perceived the risks involved. Other advisors and students at the gymnasium, once I apprised them of the plan, reiterated Dr Orser's fears. Should Belarusians organize and effectively defend the district against the Red Guerrillas, then the Eskadron could be the first step towards attaining national independence. However, once that occurred and the Germans retreated from the area, the Soviets could launch another reign of terror and subject our people to fearsome atrocities. Ultimately, we could not rely on continued German support, nor could we live independently under Soviet rule. We would struggle alone.

I reported to Commissar Traub the next day and accepted his offer. He informed me that he had arranged for me to fly to Minsk for a meeting with von Gottberg, who, after the defeat of the German army in Stalingrad, had taken office in Minsk. And so the next morning I was on a plane to Minsk in the company of a German fighter pilot and the commissar's secretary. It was the first time I had seen Minsk from the air, and the sight broke my heart. Much of the city lay in ruins. The bombers had done their work. We landed, and German soldiers were on hand to escort us to the governor general's office. Von Gottberg, with his military bearing, fine features, and intelligent eyes, impressed me. I noted the SS insignia on his uniform. Cursory introductions were made and the general reviewed the proposal for the formation of an armed cavalry force. I told him that I needed two weeks to organize a suitable unit and that within a month – if the necessary horses and equipment had been delivered – the Eskadron would be ready for active duty. Von Gottberg seemed surprised by my self-assurance, so I explained to him that we already had many students in military training in anticipation of the day their community would need defending. We discussed planning details, and I pressed von Gottberg for guarantees that the Eskadron would encounter no interference from the local authorities. I left the meeting satisfied that the project would move forward in accordance with the terms we had agreed upon.

With little time to waste, I contacted several experienced military men in the area: Lieutenant Drucko, a cavalry surgeon from the Polish army; Lieutenant Matysiak, an infantryman whose specialty was machine-gunnery; and my good friend Lieutenant Siwko, who had trained in the Polish army. I chose Siwko as my second-in-command. Each lieutenant would command a platoon, and each platoon, composed of four units, would be supplied with machine guns. Training of a small artillery unit would have to wait until I could find a suitable instructor. Within a week, we had 150 men ready to join the Belarusian Eskadron. Our soldiers wore grey German uniforms with the Belarusian insignia (a double cross) and the red-and-white flag emblazoned on the collars and sleeves.

News of the formation of the Belarusian Eskadron invoked mixed emotions among the citizens of the district. Idealistic young people viewed it as a symbol of hope that we would one day have an independent Belarusian state; others, scarred by war, believed that our valiant efforts would have no impact on the outcome of the raging conflict. One night one of my closet supporters taught me about torment and conflicting interests. He came to me to ask permission to join the Red Guerrillas because his family was being held hostage in their village. I could see that this decision was agonizing for him, so I permitted him to resign from the Eskadron. Before he left he said that he sincerely believed that what we were doing was not for Germany but for Belarus. He knew this in his heart because if I had been a German puppet, then I would not have allowed him to go back to his family. We parted as friends, and I never saw him again.

About two weeks after the organization of the Eskadron we received notification that General Helle was coming from Minsk on von Gottberg's behalf to inspect our troops, our barracks, and the exercise and drill programs. We prepared for his visit, and when he arrived I acted as his guide and interpreter. On the drill fields Helle watched the units operate with keen interest, sometimes asking for clarification, and he made a point of meeting with each of the officers. Back in the encampment he complimented us on achieving so much in such a short time, confiding that when he had visited similar units organized by the gendarmes he had found them in a state of disorganization. With pride I explained that our soldiers believed in an independent Belarusian state, and their skills derived from their commitment, discipline, and faith in the future. Helle responded to my glowing commentary by suggesting that a German officer be assigned to the Eskadron to facilitate better cooperation and communication. Bristling inwardly, I told him that our agreement with von Gottberg hinged on the unit's autonomy in all matters, but his only reply was to assure me that our supplies would arrive shortly.

Although we had made a promising start, we soon received news that threatened the success of the Eskadron. Some members of the Red Guerrillas were harassing families with sons in the Eskadron, and although no deaths had been reported, we had no doubt that the terrifying harassment would continue. Morale among the Eskadron recruits plummeted. I gathered the commanding officers to discuss the problem and to get their ideas about how we should respond. Some wanted to retaliate in kind; others spoke about negotiating a truce. In the end, however, I decided to deal with it myself. As I had no desire to persecute innocent families or instill fear in the local population, I sent a message to the guerrillas through an emissary. In it I pointed out that the Eskadron and the Red Guerrillas had a common enemy in the Germans and declared that, as commanding officer of the Eskadron, I would protect all Belarusian families in the territory, including those with members among the guerrillas. In return I wanted the Red Guerrillas to stop molesting the families in my jurisdiction. This resulted in a truce – there were no clashes between the Eskadron and the Red Guerrillas in the Navahrudak region for the duration of the war.

As a fledgling independent military unit, the Eskadron faced several challenges, from within its own ranks and from without. Although all Eskadron recruits were educated and had a good knowledge of the country's political problems, a few behaved inappropriately. In one case, some recruits were exercising near a small village, and one demanded brandy from a farmer. When the commanding officer learned of this infringement of our strict code of discipline, the soldier received one week in prison and a strong reprimand from me. If we hoped to gain support for the Eskadron, then we could show no tolerance for this sort of conduct.

One day a young man of about eighteen appeared in my office. He looked frantic, and I was immediately convinced that he had a serious problem of a personal nature. I asked my secretary and some soldiers who were on hand to leave the room. I offered the young fellow a cigarette and he declined, but he did accept a cup of strong coffee. Slowly, he relaxed enough to tell me his story. His name was Boris H. He was from Dziatlowa, and he was working on one of the collective farms now operated by the Germans when the Polish AK (Resistance) arrived and pressured the gendarme in attendance to replace some of the Belarusian employees with Polish workers. Rather than wait for the gendarme to confer with the mayor of Dziatlowa, the AK agents resorted to underhanded tactics.

They spread a rumour that Boris H. worked for the Red Guerrillas, and as soon as Boris heard of this false accusation he had no choice but to flee. When he had concluded his story, I called in the superintendent of the troops and informed him that Boris H. would now be with the Eskadron. As a member of our small company, perhaps Boris H. would have hope of a better future.

Two days later two gendarmes appeared at the gates of our encampment with orders to arrest our newest recruit. I sent them back to their headquarters with a firm message for their superior: I alone had authority in the jurisdiction of the Eskadron; since Boris H. was under my command, only I could decide his fate. Then I informed my personnel that if Commissar Traub phoned, I, and no one else, would take the call. Traub never called.

Anti-Semitism, in all its loathsome forms, did exist in Belarus. There was even a Belarusian Nazi Party (which ultimately failed to gain widespread support for German policies). However, the majority of Belarusians demonstrated a subtle passive resistance towards the unsavoury German directives. Organizations like the Belarusian Independence Party (BNP) and various youth groups and cultural clubs found ways to undermine or sabotage German acts of aggression by providing false documents, publishing illegal journals, or hiding victims.

In the Navahrudak district a number of Jews lived peacefully with other citizens. Then, in early December 1941, the German occupying forces started rounding them up on the pretext that, as artisans, they had the skills required to increase production of manufactured goods for the troops on the eastern front. When Traub took me to Germany in 1942, I learned what these enforced labour campaigns meant for Jews and other "undesirables." Many Belarusian Jews went into hiding to escape deportation or the work camps, but others ended up living in barracks under heavy German guard. Local people tried to help them by smuggling food and other necessities into the ghetto. Two of my schoolmates – Abramowicz, the girl who had helped me get my identity papers after I returned home, and Adek Levin – ended up in the barracks. Adek believed, falsely, that as long as the captive workforce served Germany's needs, the Jews would be safe. In August 1943 his hopes were brutally dashed. Residents of Navahrudak were ordered to stay off the streets and to keep their windows and curtains closed. A group of perhaps 300 Jews from the barracks were then marched through the downtown district, Abramowicz among them. We heard rumours that the Germans had transported the Jews by truck to another village, but it later seemed more likely that they executed these people and buried them in mass graves.

Adek came to see me shortly afterwards, and I could see his pain and fear, but I could neither confirm nor deny the rumours. I urged him to make his escape from the ghetto and join the partisan guerrillas. I offered to get a message to Victor's unit through Mrs Hutor. Uncertainty clouding his reason, Adek left me saying he would have to think it over. During this time of escalating persecution against the Jews, the Germans brought battalions from the Estonian army to Navahrudak. Officially these troops had orders to join in the fight against the Red Army. I invited Eric, their young captain, to my apartment for a meal. After a few glasses of vodka and some *zakuska*, we started talking freely about our political views. We quickly discovered that we shared fears and hopes for the liberation of our homelands. Several days later Eric came to visit me again. By now he knew the real reason for his battalion's transfer to Navahrudak. The Germans wanted to proceed more rapidly with their "final solution" to the "Jewish problem" and needed help with their barbaric mission. Eric, visibly distressed, vowed to me that he would not let his men dirty their hands by executing Jews. Although his position was tenuous, we agreed to work together to undermine the Germans' sinister program.

Some days later Adek again sought me out. He announced that he intended to escape and then, exhausted by pent-up fear and misery, he sat in silence, tears streaming down his face. I took his hand, but I could offer no words of comfort. I did, however, ask friends at City Hall to prepare a false passport and travel documents for him. After laying the groundwork through the BNP network, I gave Adek Mrs Hutor's address and a verbal message. I knew that Victor would accept Adek into his troop. I never saw Adek again. Sometimes, when I look back on those days, I am haunted by shadowy memories of lost friends.

At the beginning of 1944, the German authorities sent a young lieutenant, Rudy, to act as chief of security in the Navahrudak district. Rudy summoned a number of citizens, among them municipal leaders and teachers, to a meeting to discuss security problems in the district. I sat at this gathering listening to Rudy talk about the future of Belarus within the Third Reich, and somehow his assertions seemed hollow. He did not speak with the same conviction and arrogance as other Nazi officers I had met. However, when he declared that he wanted us to provide him with information about certain local groups and individuals, I felt embittered. Without a word, I stood up, put on my coat, and walked out. I would not spy for the Germans. Rudy followed me out the door, imploring me to give him a chance to explain his position, and his tone and his words took the edge off my anger and disappointment. He alerted me to the gendarmes' plans to have me removed from Navahrudak and warned me that I was being followed, urging me to be wary. If the Germans uncovered any proof of my collaboration with the partisan guerrillas, he could not protect me. As proof of his sincerity, he showed me a crumpled note that he had found on a guerrilla who had died during a raid by the gendarmes. Fortunately, Rudy had been the first person to search this man, and no one else knew about the note. Skeptics might think that Rudy had orchestrated all of this merely to gain my trust, but as I look back on our relationship, I still remember him as a humane and compassionate person.

One spring day we had wonderful news. The Jews had escaped from the ghetto! They had tunnelled under the fence, and with the help of local sympathizers they had joined the partisan guerrillas. The older people and the highly skilled craftsmen stayed behind, and, surprisingly, the Germans left them in peace.

While members of the BNP and the local network of Belarusian patriots continued to work towards achieving independence, we learned of promising developments in Minsk. Governor General von Gottberg had called Professor Ostrowski, a former director of the Polish gymnasium in Vilnius during the Polish regime, to Minsk during the early part of 1943, and he had instructed him to organize a Belarusian Central Rada (council). This body had no significant administrative power, and many Belarusians perceived its creation as just another ploy to bolster their allegiance to the Germans, but when I met Ostrowski I sensed that he shared our dream of an independent Belarus. Executives of the BNP discussed the Rada and its potential for promoting our cause, and BNP agents were gradually able to infiltrate the Rada's administrative structures. I suspected that Ostrowski tacitly approved of the activities of the Belarusian underground, because in the spring of 1943 he asked me to be the Rada's representative in Navahrudak. My colleagues and I carefully gauged the implications of such an involvement. According to Rudy, German authorities and the local gendarmes were actively seeking means to eliminate me. By accepting the public role of Rada regional representative, I would be even more vulnerable, but despite the risks I accepted the appointment.

In April 1943 von Gottberg stepped up plans for organizing a Belarusian army. Since the guerrillas' presence in the area threatened the Germans' mobilization of local troops, the occupying forces enlisted the Eskadron to help with the selection and mobilization of recruits. When the Eskadron arrived in the area near Lubcza and Kareliczy, the local German gendarmes suggested that our two companies work together. However, one of my men, Lieutenant K., refused to do this because it would violate the Eskadron's autonomy in regional defence matters. The gendarmes conceded and proceeded to work in another area. Our recruitment went smoothly until an Eskadron unit arrived in Delatyczy and local guerrillas opened fire on them. Lieutenant K. quickly deployed the troops under his command, dispersed the guerrillas, and captured one young man. When the gendarmes came upon the scene, their commander announced that he would take the prisoner into custody and decide his fate. The leader of the Eskadron detachment, Sergeant D., stood his ground and insisted that the prisoner was the responsibility of his unit. Grudgingly, the gendarme commander backed down. Then Sergeant D. approached the terrified young man, who was only about nineteen years old. The fellow stated his name and explained that the Red Guerrillas had come to his village. Soon after they left, a German unit overran the village, executed many residents, and razed the buildings. With nowhere else to go, the young man had joined the partisan guerrillas – like so many others, he had done so to save himself because the German forces had badly mismanaged the situation in Belarus. Sergeant D. told the prisoner that the Eskadron were not the Germans, nor were they enemies of their fellow countrymen; they were there to protect Belarusians not only from the Germans, but also from the Red Guerrillas. He then told the lad that he could either join the Eskadron or go back to the partisan guerrillas. Fear and disbelief washed over his face, and he looked frantically from Sergeant D. to the commander of the gendarmes. He turned and bolted into the wooded area bordering the village. When the commander ordered his men to surround the village and burn it to the ground, Sergeant D. counter-ordered the Eskadron to take up positions against the would-be raiders. The gendarmes retreated. The villagers, who had observed the confrontation, flooded into the market square and carried members of the Eskadron into their homes, calling them "angels sent by God." News of this event spread rapidly through the countryside. By defying the gendarmes and refusing to adopt tactics of terror and destruction, the Eskadron had won the hearts of Belarusians. When I learned of this incident, I was convinced that our fledgling Belarusian army could uphold the ideals of justice.

Confrontations of this nature continually challenged leaders of the Eskadron to rely on peaceful negotiations rather than armed force. In March 1944, our company received intelligence that the Polish underground army, the AK, had crossed the Nieman River and taken up positions in an abandoned glass factory on Belarusian territory. Some members of my staff demanded immediate action to oust the AK and assert our territorial rights. When this happened I was preparing to go to Minsk to see Colonel Kushel, a high-ranking member of the BNP who wanted to send me to Vilnius to meet with a representative of the Polish government and proceed with sensitive discussions concerning the possibility of a political alliance between the Poles and Belarusians.[1] Before I left on this important mission, I met with Lieutenant Siwko, my second-in-command. We agreed that the Eskadron would make every effort to avoid an armed confrontation with the AK because, like us, the Polish underground army received equipment and weapons from the Germans, and the Germans would enjoy seeing us pitted against one another – infighting would only weaken us.

An Eskadron detachment led by Siwko approached the glass factory, and three Polish soldiers emerged bearing a white flag, a signal that the Poles also sought a peaceful resolution. The Polish contingent escorted Siwko and three other members of the Eskadron to a meeting near the village of Huta. No one carried weapons. In the mid-afternoon, Siwko and the Polish commander, Captain Roger, met. Siwko spoke frankly, explaining that the Eskadron knew that the Germans supplied arms and equipment to the AK in order to secure the Polish army's help in fighting the Red Guerrillas. He went on to describe several military skirmishes that had resulted in the needless deaths of innocent Belarusian civilians in the area surrounding Lida. In the Navahrudak region, continued Siwko, people of Polish descent lived without fear of persecution from either the local population or the Eskadron. In defence of the Polish army's activities, Captain Roger said that the nature of guerrilla warfare inevitably created problems for both the high command and the local inhabitants. He gave Siwko his promise as a military officer that he would do everything possible to curtail unprovoked attacks by his guerrillas, but Siwko insisted that he also communicate the situation to his superiors. The demoralizing effects of the attacks against civilians in the Belarusian territory had to be considered by those with the power and authority to change the military objectives of the AK.

After this intense and lengthy conference, Siwko and Roger shared a drink and parted on good terms. At the end of the day, Siwko watched soldiers take down the Polish flag. The Polish troops assembled, crossed the Nieman River, and entered Lida territory. Once the dust had settled, Siwko's men hoisted the Belarusian flag. When I learned of this masterful piece of negotiation, I knew that Siwko and other like-minded officers of the Eskadron had the potential to bring peace and order to our homeland.

While Siwko was dealing with the Polish problem on the Nieman River, I was in Minsk meeting with Colonel Kushel. From there I travelled to Vilnius, where I was met by three gentlemen who were supposedly representing the Polish government and living in exile in England. I spoke to them of the need for the Polish AK and Belarusian forces to work for a common cause. The Polish envoys responded by citing the difficulties of managing and controlling guerrilla troops, but they assured me that they would strive to avoid future conflicts. As our meeting progressed, I learned from them that the British government and the Soviet Union had formed an alliance. Although the envoys understood the goals of the Belarusian people, they could not provide official support for our anti-Soviet activities, given the recent political alliance with the Western Allies. Once again I realized that many in the Western world misunderstood the question of Belarusian independence – or, worse still, they did not consider it a factor in global political developments. The Polish envoys believed that Poland would one day achieve independence and that British, American, and Soviet powers would sanction Poland's national integrity. Belarus was not on the agenda.

I returned to Minsk and gave a full report to Colonel Kushel. Neither of us felt that much had been accomplished; we clearly lacked the power to influence the Allied powers' policies. Back in Navahrudak, I received a call from Rudy. He had heard about the incident at the glass factory and my trip to Vilnius. When I expressed surprise at his knowledge of my movements, he told me that many people were watching me and reporting on my activities. I took this as a warning.

As commander of the Eskadron, I often had conflicts with the local German gendarmes. In March one of my officers, Lieutenant Drucko, had a falling out with a gendarme and dared to hit the man. For this he was sent to prison in Navahrudak. I used my authority to free him, and then I promoted him to the position of officer in command of cavalry instruction. This was a calculated risk – my aim was to bolster Belarusian support for the Eskadron. On 25 March, the anniversary of the 1918 Declaration of Independence, members of the Eskadron were scheduled to take their public oath of allegiance to Belarus. Some Navahrudak women embroidered insignia for our uniforms depicting the Belarusian national emblem and colours, and organizers arranged for the ceremony to take place on the grounds of the old Belarusian castle. Hundreds of men, women, and children attended. Three soldiers from every unit of the Eskadron came forward and swore allegiance to the Belarusian ideal of independence, vowing to fight to the death for it. The Belarusian national anthem rang out loud and clear. After the ceremony the teachers' college opened its doors to the community.

We danced and ate and sang, and for a short time we escaped the turmoil of the world around us.

Meanwhile, mobilization and recruitment of troops for a Belarusian army proceeded at a steady pace, but not without some difficulties. In the town of Kareliczy, Eskadron Sergeant M., a former student of the University of Vilnius, arranged several meetings with representatives of the partisan guerrillas. Most of these guerrillas, considered Communists by the Polish government, believed that the Communist regime would allow an independent Belarus. Under the noses of the local German gendarmes, our troops smuggled several influential guerrilla leaders to meetings with me in Navahrudak. While we, the Eskadron, shared political goals with the guerrillas, they operated under different command structures. Guerrilla leaders working out of Moscow primarily used their networks to fight the Germans, not to attain national independence for Belarus. Most of the guerrillas conceded that the Soviet Union had failed to support or sanction independent republics in the past and that it was unlikely that the Communists would now make dramatic policy changes. Like so many other resistance groups, the guerrillas found themselves mired in wartime politics. At the secret Navahrudak meetings I attempted to establish clearly articulated roles for the Eskadron and the partisan guerrillas, but I cannot claim to have succeeded. At best, the Eskadron remained a symbol of hope for Belarusian nationalists.

By the spring of 1944 the Eskadron's ranks had swollen to 450. We now occupied the barracks at Skydlevo, an excellent training facility about three kilometres from Navahrudak. It was during this intensive mobilization that I decided to step down as the Rada's representative in Navahrudak. Mr Ostrowski, although very persuasive and committed to his public role as the representative of the Belarusian people, had not managed to gain any administrative powers. Without a political voice, I decided to concentrate my efforts on the training and expansion of the Eskadron. Soon the Eskadron would have to prove its mettle.

Sometime in April the Eskadron received supplies of weaponry and ammunition. Shortly thereafter I discovered through our intelligence networks that Commander Micka, leader of the Red Guerrillas in the Kareliczy area, was boasting of his unit's superior manpower and ability to eliminate the Eskadron. Determined to demonstrate the strength of the Eskadron to civilians in the outlying areas, I devised a plan with my officers. We knew that if we remained cloistered in Navahrudak the guerrillas would continue to terrorize innocent people and discredit us, so we mounted a sojourn into guerrilla-infested areas. We were prepared for a fight. Our first stops would be Lake Switez and the village of Parecza, then we would move on to Haradyszcza, another guerrilla stronghold. Next, our route would take us through Palaneczka, Mir, Turec, Kareliczy, and Zabalocie, a veritable Red Guerrilla headquarters. On 28 April, cheered on by the citizens of Navahrudak, we set out. As we rode away people called out their good wishes and bid us a speedy and safe return.

We travelled in routine military order, with patrols at the front, rear, and flanks. Just as we were approaching Switez, one of the patrols brought an old man to me. He bore a stark warning message from the Red Guerrillas: leave the area or die. Stifling my misgivings, I smiled at the messenger and told him to return to the guerrilla leaders with our reply: this was Belarusian territory, protected by the Eskadron. My commanders and I consulted, and we decided to inform the troops of the heavy guerrilla presence. Not one man faltered – each understood that this public display of strength was necessary to the future success of the Eskadron. And so we proceeded. On the road to Haradyszcza our patrols reported sightings of guerrilla detachments moving parallel to our unit. I ordered them to continue to report any guerrilla activity.

We dismounted at the edge of the forest and walked to the shore of Lake Switez, where we watered the horses and took a little time to rest before continuing on to Parecza. As we entered that village, my heart churned in anguish. The guerrillas had torched it. Parecza was no longer a thriving village – it was a wasteland. We surveyed the damage, found no survivors, and continued our march.

At Haradyszcza, our mood lightened. Raising their voices in a song of welcome, the inhabitants invited us into their homes for refreshments. I ordered perimeter guards to patrol the area while the rest of the troops enjoyed a brief respite from the march. Officers and soldiers alike told the townspeople the purpose of our mission. One skeptical citizen pointed out that we, the Eskadron, demonstrated national enthusiasm and ideals, but we lacked reason – how could such a small force expect to play any great part in the war between the superpowers? I responded by reiterating the idealistic philosophy of the Eskadron and other patriots who fought for an independent Belarus. Despite the strength and number of our enemies, I insisted, we would preserve our history and fight for our future by promoting and protecting Belarusian ideals. Many people nodded their heads in agreement, and hundreds began to pray: "God help you. Bless those who believe." The despair and suffering of these people were vivid to me in this moment. The times were uncertain, and their hope was so fragile.

As evening drew near, the local commander of the German gendarmes came into town to speak with me. He warned me that all the villages in the area lay in guerrilla territory, and the gendarmes could not protect our troops. He seemed annoyed when I explained that we had set out on this mission fully aware that we could only depend on our own forces, that we had not asked for, nor did we expect, their assistance. At dawn on the following day, we made ready to leave Haradyszcza. Our next destination was Mir, by way of Palaneczka and Zuhwiczy. We reviewed our defensive strategies, and we all agreed that there would be no retreat if we encountered armed resistance. In Palaneczka, we saw smouldering rubble. Our front patrols started to sing a popular Belarusian song to alert any survivors that we came in peace, and the streets gradually filled with people who pointed to our insignia with obvious relief. We learned that a band of well-armed Red Guerrillas, or perhaps Germans, had rampaged through the town and that many of the townspeople had died of burns or other injuries; others had fled and taken refuge in nearby wooded areas. Women brought baskets of food and drink for us, but I told them to save it for themselves – it was enough that they considered us "sons of a true Belarus."

At the end of this tiring and sobering day we arrived in Mir, once an internationally renowned center for horse training. Before the war, German, French, Italian, and Dutch horse breeders had travelled here to acquire the best breeding stock in Europe. One of Mir's major historical and architectural attractions was Mir Castle, which dated to 1495. News of our arrival spread through the town, and the castle's owner – an elderly prince of the aristocratic Mirski family – invited us to visit him. During our visit, this engaging and astute member of the deposed aristocracy asked me many questions about the purpose of the Eskadron and the various unruly political factions of the day. Speaking about Belarusian statehood, he expressed regret that the country's aristocracy had blithely joined the ranks of the Polish and Russian intelligentsia with the hope of gaining influence and status. I realized that this man, and others of his generation, had seen their life circumstances, their belief systems, and their ideals torn apart by unforeseen foreign events. I had no words to console the old prince.

Later in the day I ordered the troops to assemble in the marketplace with a newly mobilized Mir battalion. As the riders passed through the square and went into formation, a cry of "Long live the battalion of Mir!" rang through the air. Mir and Eskadron commanders made inspiring speeches, but they also stated the current political situation clearly. Bolshevik Communists had no intention of granting independence to our small nation. The Western democracies were now allied with the USSR, and Germany's power in the area was rapidly diminishing. Belarusians had to rely on their patriotic sons to win political freedom and autonomy for them. There was hope in the faces of the rallying civilians. An explosion of applause and many gestures of support for our cause brought sunshine into the square. Indeed, it was one of the best days of our march.

We left Mir and headed towards Turec on 29 April. There, in my birthplace, many of my father's friends welcomed the Eskadron. A number of them came to me with their memories and stories of my father, telling me how skilled and caring he had been in his work. I tried to suppress the emotions these stories inspired in me. I thought my voice would break if I attempted to speak, and I had to maintain the demeanour of a military commander.

The Turec police outlined for us the dangers we would face along the road from Turec to Kareliczy. Micka, a fearsome partisan guerrilla leader, had effectively cut off communications between the two towns. At the river crossing near Kareliczy, which was located in an open area, our troops would be most vulnerable. Armed with this information, I assembled the battalion leaders so that we could review our strategy. We ordered the Eskadron to avoid armed conflict and to camouflage their machine-gun positions. Early into the march from Turec the patrols reported sightings of the guerrillas. The first platoons reached the river-crossing point without incident and set to work installing the machine guns and digging trenches to defend their comrades who were still en route to this meeting place. The situation remained tense but peaceful until the second platoon made its attempt to cross the river. The Kareliczy police hammered them with machine-gun fire, thinking that they were Red Guerrillas. There were some frantic communications, and finally the Kareliczy forces allowed us to cross the river and enter the town. The police chief made arrangements for our men and horses to rest and eat.

During the Eskadron's second night in Kareliczy, I assigned troops to guard the barracks housing the new, unarmed recruits. Under cover of darkness, three guerrillas broke into our encampment and opened fire on the guards. One guard, Sergeant K., sustained a head injury, and as he struggled with his attackers he was blinded by the blood flowing into his eyes. He managed to lay his hand on a grenade, and he pulled the pin. He died instantly, but he took the three guerrillas with him, thereby saving the lives of the young recruits. The incident induced anger and despair among the troops, but the townspeople hailed us as heroes.

Not long after the guerrilla attack the mayor of Kareliczy organized a reception for the Eskadron leaders in order to introduce us to his administrators. Our hosts proclaimed their support for our recruitment efforts; and in anticipation of an Allied victory over Germany, the mayor advised all who were able to go west. He maintained that the Western democracies would not long tolerate Stalin's rule by terror and deprivation and that the USSR would soon find itself politically ostracized. Some of the administrators warned that our plan to proceed through guerrilla-controlled areas would result in many casualties and discourage potential recruits from joining our unit. Nonetheless, I conferred with my battalion leaders, and we decided to proceed with the next segment of our operation. We would enlist the help of the Kareliczy police – they would march in the direction of Raviny, Rutkavicy, and Zareca, drawing the Red Guerrilla forces to this area while the Eskadron set up positions along the ravines on the northwestern perimeter of Rutkavicy. We would thus encircle the guerrillas and be able to take their headquarters. But, as we would later discover, an informer within the Kareliczy police had alerted the enemy.

Before daylight the next morning the police detachment and the Eskadron set out from Kareliczy. The guerrillas, familiar with the terrain, had the upper hand. Scaling the steep, overgrown ravines hauling heavy canon and other weaponry, we lost precious time. A messenger brought news that the police detachment had reached Rutkavicy without encountering any resistance, but when Eskadron troops reached this village, I began to suspect trouble. We decided to send a well-armed detachment to Zabalocie, Zarecce, and Tupaly with Lieutenant Siwko in command. Siwko soon reported back to us that two large bands of guerrillas were heading towards Tupaly and Paluzza. The guerrillas were now in a position to encircle us. I gave the order to hold fire because I did not want to disclose our positions. Other patrols reported another large band of guerrillas taking up positions on our rear flank, cutting off our retreat to Kareliczy. With little time to manoeuvre, we moved men and armaments to the top of the ravine overlooking Kareliczy. Guerrillas rapidly appeared at the foot of the ravine. Although the guerrilla forces outnumbered the Eskadron, their troops dispersed in response to our barrage of gunfire. Siwko brought his men to our right flank just as the guerrillas started to attack our front lines. Our heavy fire once again broke the guerrilla lines and forced a retreat. Eskadron troops held the top of the ravine, but Lieutenant Drucko was caught with his squad at the bottom of the ravine. He quickly assessed the situation and ordered his men to climb straight up the side of the ravine with their mounts. Although this seemed physically impossible, they somehow made it to their target position. When I had a chance to reconnoitre, I saw blood pouring from a nasty wound on Drucko's leg. He refused to dismount or move to the rear because the next wave of guerrillas was fast approaching. By deploying the heavy machine guns and grenade throwers, we managed to break the guerrilla lines. However, some guerrilla fighters continued their upward climb to our position, so we continued to fire on them, filling the air with smoke and noise. By about five o'clock in the afternoon, the guerrilla forces had started a disorganized but steady retreat. I ordered my men to assemble in formation, with patrols on all sides. We were heading back to Kareliczy.

The mayor and a crowd of supporters came out to meet us. We buried one of our soldiers and mourned the loss of four others, who had apparently been taken prisoner by the guerrillas. Despite these losses, we believed that we had accomplished our goal and proven that the Eskadron could protect its territory. After a few days of rest we started the long trek home to Navahrudak. Along the way we heard rumours that the Eskadron had been wiped out. I could only imagine what effect these stories had had on our loved ones. I thought of Ludmila, and my heart ached.

On the first day of May the citizens of Navahrudak gathered to celebrate Labour Day. When the commissar took the podium to launch the festivities, someone shouted, "The Eskadron are coming!" People flew out of the market square to greet us, and no one looked back at the German commissar and his administrators. Our return became the focus of the celebration. Our supporters arranged for food, stabling for the horses, and medical care, and they even organized a dance at the teachers' college. In the milling, happy crowd, I found Ludmila and blurted out a proposal of marriage. She turned me down, explaining that she wanted to graduate from high school first. Her graduation would take place in June. I could wait.

Since the recruitment program had increased our ranks, sections of the Eskadron moved to other command posts. Most of the senior men became commanders in the newly formed battalions. However, I managed to maintain a unit of thirty men for the defense of Navahrudak. While this reorganization of the Eskadron took place, the BNP made plans to meet in Minsk on 27 June. Rodzko, the leader of the BNP, came to Navahrudak because he wanted my battalion to guard the Rada. He also wanted to discuss with me his plan to depose the German commissar, which would open the way for the Rada to declare independence for Belarus. I balked at this because it would amount to a total denunciation of the Germans and the Soviets, and Soviet troops still controlled an area about 200 kilometres east of Minsk. As the Soviets advanced westward more innocent people would be persecuted and terrorized by the Communist forces. By a stroke of fate, the German authorities ordered me to take my unit to Dokszycy, where the main force of the Soviet guerrillas had broken through the lines. Once the guerrilla units had been dispersed, the Eskadron could go on to Minsk to guard the Rada delegates. I felt torn. Was this some sort of elaborate German scheme to remove me from the area? Was Rodzko using the Eskadron as bait? I had deep misgivings, but I agreed to support the Rada.

When we arrived in Dokszycy, we saw signs of Red Guerrilla and German savagery everywhere. Chimneys rose from the ruins of homes and businesses, stark witnesses to the horror, destruction, and human suffering. Nothing had escaped the hail of bullets and the raging fires. My unit took up positions on the western edge of the marshlands and awaited the next guerrilla attack. Our patrols sighted straggling guerrilla patrols, but we did not engage them. Empty days passed with no sign of the enemy. By 25 June our troops had become restless and anxious. Sensing the approach of the Soviets, they wanted to return home to their families and decide whether to retreat to the West or stay and face the unknown. I shared their preoccupations and longed to be in Navahrudak. Now, as I look back on this futile exercise, I have a lingering suspicion that the Eskadron was being used as a decoy. We had no information about events occurring beyond our small territory, and so it was instinct that eventually compelled us homeward. On 2 July, on our approach to Navahrudak, we saw many civilians fleeing their homes to escape the impending onslaught of the Red Army. We stayed our course, haunted by the fear we saw in the faces of our fellow citizens.

In the early-morning hours of 3 July 1944 we reached our destination. Navahrudak was a practically ghost town. At the Eskadron barracks a few soldiers were still holding their posts, and I impressed upon them the danger of the situation. I urged them to decide whether to stay or retreat within the next twenty-four hours, and one asked me what the West had to offer. I had to tell him that I did not know, but that under a Soviet regime one could expect long years in enforced labour camps, or death. I left my troops and went to find Ludmila.

At the Hutor home everyone was still asleep. I roused them, and they were shocked to see that I was alive. In Ludmila's eyes I saw relief and what I hoped was love for me. Again I asked her to marry me, this time vowing that I would not leave without her. Then I asked her mother and father for their blessing. With tears trickling down her face, Mrs Hutor told me that she trusted me to care for her daughter, and with a warm hug, she consented. She gave Ludmila a fur coat and said it was to keep her warm and to remind her that her parents were praying for her safety. Mr Hutor said little, but he was obviously deeply moved. We shook hands and embraced, and he told me to take good care of his daughter. I assured them both that I would do everything in my power to protect Ludmila and care for her.

A few hours later I went to speak with a priest, but he refused to marry us. He explained that it was a time of fasting before a religious holiday and no marriages could take place in the church. Summoning up all my powers of persuasion, I begged him to reconsider because Ludmila and I had to leave for the West. In dogmatic fashion, he blessed our journey but still refused to perform the marriage ceremony. I had to control the anger and frustration welling up inside me. While it meant little to me, I knew that Ludmila would be distressed if we were not married by a priest. But in the end we had no choice – we were married in a civil ceremony at City Hall. There was no time to celebrate because reports came in that the Red Army was only twenty kilometres from Navahrudak. I left Ludmila to pack her things, and I returned to my unit. There

I released the remaining soldiers from duty so that those who chose to retreat could do so with a clear conscience.

The next morning Ludmila and I said our farewells to her family. Janka had decided to come with us (although he had to leave his girlfriend, Taisa, behind), and I implored Mr and Mrs Hutor to do the same, but Mrs Hutor insisted that she had to stay and care for her other children. Besides, Mr Hutor refused to leave; if he had to suffer and die, he said, then he would do it in his homeland. As we parted, they wished us luck and told us to remain faithful to the ideals of Belarus.

We were on the brink of our departure when Rudy came to see me. He was clearly anxious and deeply troubled, and he asked me to perform one last service for him. The Germans had ordered him to the eastern front, and he doubted that he would ever see his home again. He asked me to go to see his mother and tell her that her son was not a Nazi. We looked at one another in silence before I found the words to comfort him. I promised him that I would do as he asked. I would describe to his mother the Rudy I knew – a man who embraced humanity and did all he could to protect innocent people. When we said goodbye, I felt an emptiness within my soul. Rudy and I never met again.[2]

From Navahrudak we headed for Lida. During the journey I struggled inwardly, tormented by the thought that perhaps all of my work had been for nothing. My friends and colleagues in the underground movement faced persecution or death if the Red Army found them. We were leaving everything behind, including our hope for a free and independent Belarus. To the Soviets we were traitors and to the Germans we were mere pawns of their imperfectly constructed empire. As we plodded on, these words of Polish poet Adam Mickiewicz lingered in my mind: "Only those who have lost their freedom know how precious it is." We finally made it to the outskirts of Lida, but the Soviet forces were attacking the city. That night we hid in the fields, but by midnight the bombing had ceased and we crept into the city to witness the destruction. Everywhere we saw misery, fear, and panic. We had no help to give, so with heavy hearts we set out for Grodno, and as we walked through the countryside I hoped that the blood of our brothers would nourish the seeds of a free and independent Belarus.

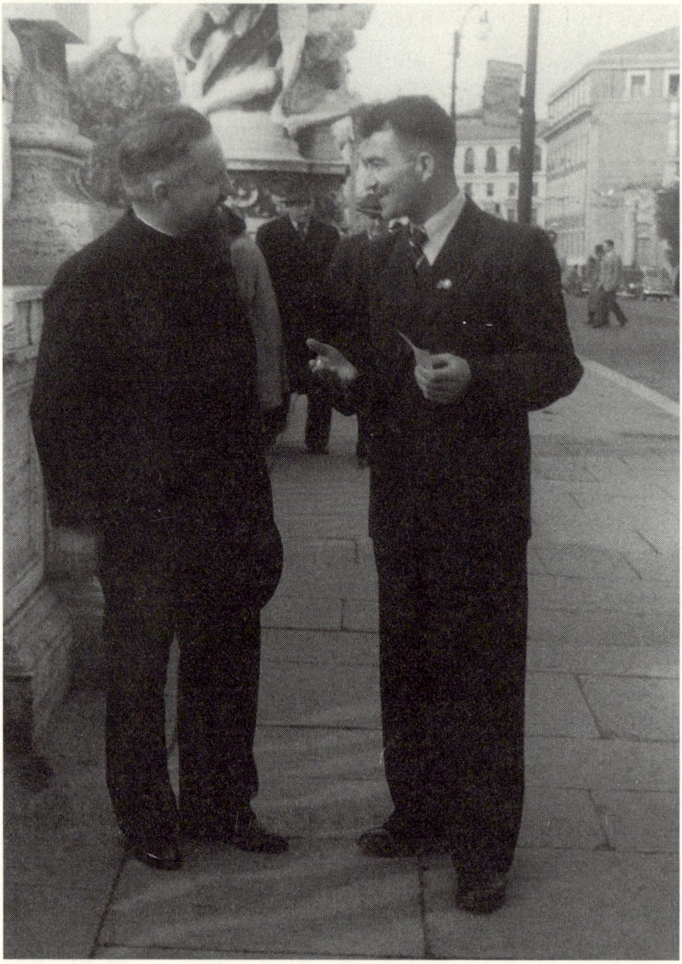

Boris and Father Robert VanCawelart, Louvain, Belgium, 1949. Using his church connections, the Benedictine monk arranged for Boris to have an audience with Pope Pius XII

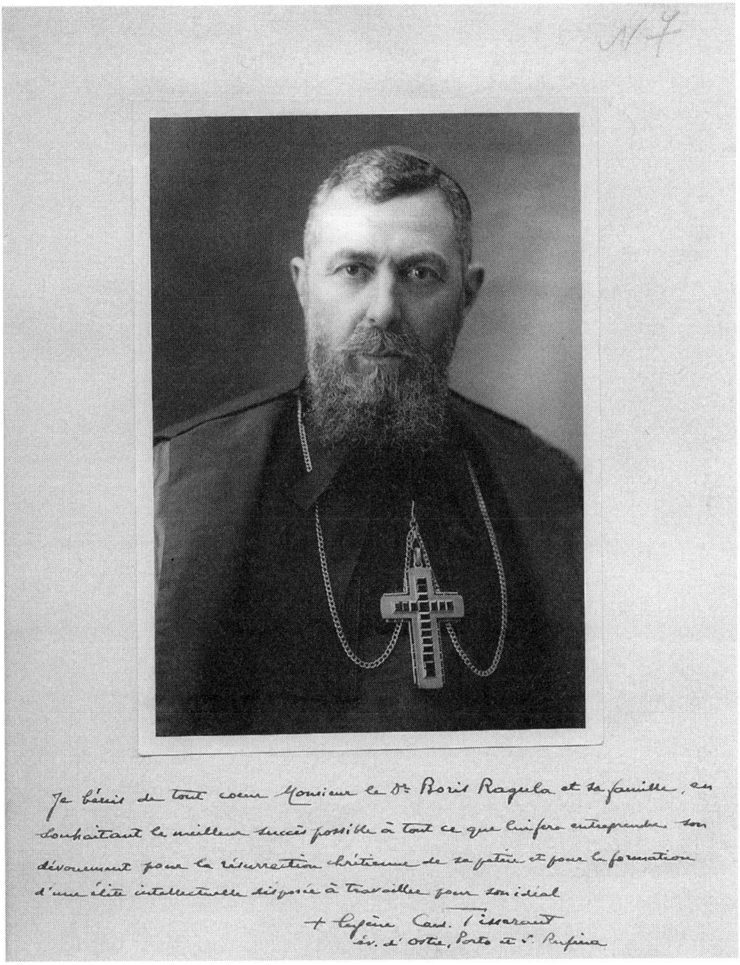

Cardinal Tisserant, c.1949. The cardinal, a high-ranking aid to Pope Pius XII, initially disapproved of Boris asking the pope for scholarships for Belarusian refugees, but soon after Boris returned to Belgium, Tisserant sent him this photograph and a personal message of encouragement

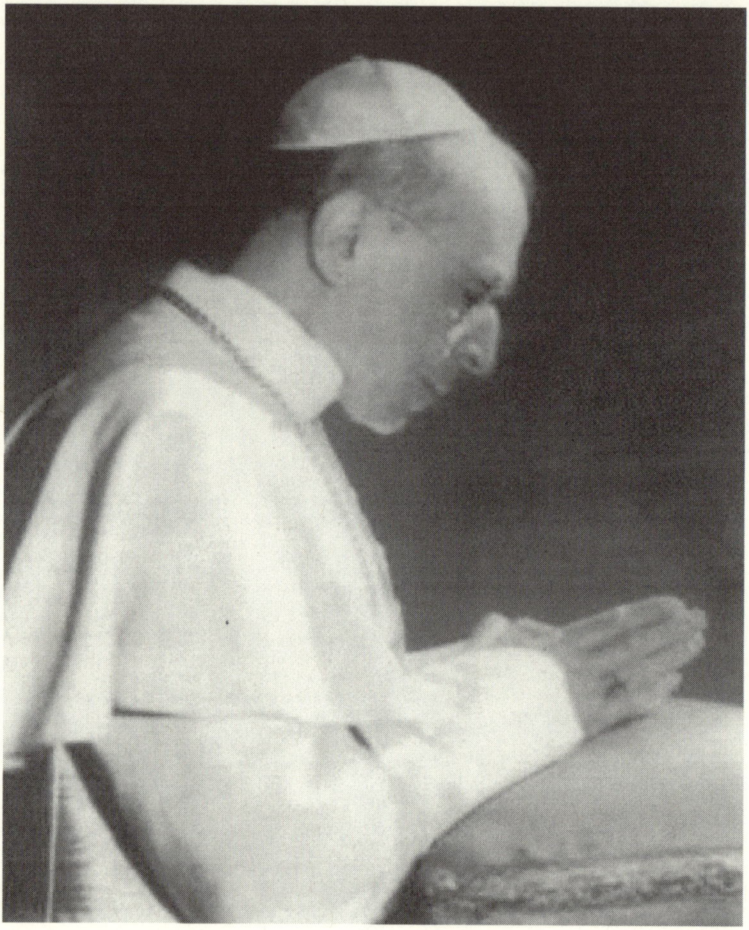

Pope Pius XII, c.1949

5 Refugees in the West

It was 5 May 1945, and suddenly everything was still. There were no booming guns, no droning bombers overhead. At last the sounds of war were silenced. Germany had surrendered to the Allies, and hundreds of thousands of people were trying to rebuild their lives.

A number of historians have examined the plight of the five million Soviets living in liberated Germany in the early post-war years.[1] Many of these refugees had fled their homeland during the war in order to escape persecution from the Red Army, and they ended up in German labour camps. Whatever their rank or status, they all faced an unwelcome repatriation. During this time Ludmila and I and a small group of Belarusians stayed in Saalfield, Thuringia, which was under American control. We were careful to hide from the American military police because if they apprehended us we would also be repatriated, and we had no illusions about what awaited us in Stalin's USSR. News about the death camps, systematic torture, deliberate starvation, and other inhumane treatment of returned prisoners did not reach the Western world until decades after the Iron Curtain fell, but we knew about life under Stalin. Consequently, when we learned that the Americans intended to leave Thuringia and allow the Soviets to occupy the territory, we scrambled to move west of the demarcation line.

Despite my sense of insecurity, I held fast to my dream of becoming a medical doctor. When I heard about the famous Philipps University in Marburg, West Germany, I resolved to go there. Accompanied by my small group I travelled to Marburg by train in early September 1945. Once we had found accommodations, I went to the medical school to try to convince the dean to allow me to start my studies. Although I did not have an appointment, the dean's secretary listened as I recounted my story, and she seemed sympathetic. She told me to wait, and after a few minutes she came and escorted me to Professor Benninghof's office. I shook the professor's hand and gave him a detailed account of my war years in Belarus. He listened patiently and then asked me what I wanted. I was a homeless Belarusian, I explained, and I was looking for some assistance from the West. I told him that my father had been a medical doctor and my mother a nurse, and I too wished to pursue a medical career. Benninghof studied me carefully. "Courses start on 15 September," he said. "You can go and register." I was so stunned and grateful that I just stood there in front of his desk gulping for air, but then I recovered my senses enough to tell him that there were fifteen others in my Belarusian group who wanted to enter the university. "All for medical school?" he asked. "No," I said, "perhaps four or five. The rest are interested in other fields." Benninghof stood up slowly and told me that he would see what he could do to help. He then instructed me to give him a list of those who sought admission and their chosen faculties. Overcome with joy and gratitude, I had to force myself not to embrace my new benefactor. Professor Benninghof shook my hand heartily and sent me on my way with wishes for our future success. I assured him that he would never regret giving us this chance to make a new life for ourselves.

Not long after this triumph, however, Ludmila and I were heartbroken by the loss of our first child. Ludmila was five months pregnant and understandably fell into a deep depression. When she recovered her health, she also enrolled in the university and began to study pharmacology. We still faced the threat of repatriation, but the Marburg Belarusian Student Organization helped us circumvent the system that would have forced many of us to return to the USSR. Some of us had certificates identifying us as Polish citizens, but others held travel documents issued by the Soviet Union, and, as Soviet citizens, these refugees were vulnerable. The student organization therefore arranged for Polish students to lease apartments for their Soviet colleagues, effectively hiding them from the authorities. By the end of 1946, however, the Allied Forces were refusing to enforce the repatriation of Soviet citizens, and such subterfuge was no longer necessary.

Through the UNRRA (United Nations Relief and Rehabilitation Administration), we received provisions and clothing, and this enabled us to survive. There was a flourishing black market in Germany, and with two packages of cigarettes one could pay tuition and rent. As long as UNRRA supplied us with cigarettes, chocolate, and coffee, we managed quite well. However, by 1948 the global political situation threatened our future prospects.[2] Clashing Soviet and American visions for post-war Germany fuelled national animosities, which were expressed in harsh ideological terms – democracy and capitalism versus communism. Berlin, which lay deep within the Soviet zone of occupation, had been divided into four zones by the Allies. When the Soviet Union demanded control of the entire city, the Western Allies refused. Western nations attempted to revive Berlin's economy in the spring of 1948, and the Soviets set up blockades on all highways, railway lines, and river routes to West Berlin in June.[3] But even with the Allies' support, many students feared the outbreak of war. A number of our group abandoned their studies and emigrated to Australia, Canada, and the United States. Ludmila and I decided that we would stay on until I completed my medical studies.

When the Americans launched the Marshall Plan, a massive European aid program designed to rebuild the shattered European economies, the black market could no longer provide refugees with a ready source of income. I was desperate to find a way to pay our tuition and living expenses. If we worked, then we could not study. While we were struggling with this problem, I met the president of Belarusians in Exile, a group that actively opposed the Soviet regime. He told me about the Catholic University of Louvain, Belgium, which had a special program for foreign students from behind the Iron Curtain. Applying for residency in Belgium through the normal channels was still risky, since many of us had invalid identification papers. To avoid bureaucratic scrutiny and the problems it would pose for us in obtaining eligibility for residency, we would have to enter Belgium illegally, procure the required travel and residency documents, and then return to Germany. I met with the other Belarusian students and outlined this plan for them, but none volunteered to go – instead, they urged me to make the trip alone! Finally, however, two of them agreed to accompany me. I was reluctant to leave Ludmila, but the other students promised they would take care of her during my absence.

In early June 1949, after I had completed my third year of medical studies, the three of us crossed the border into Belgium. We knew that if the authorities arrested us, then we would serve three months in prison and face deportation; but we considered it a risk worth taking. Fortunately, we entered Belgium without incident and boarded a train to Liège. There we met a friend, also a Belarusian refugee, who lent us money and helped us find work in a Louvain steel factory. As I toiled in that factory I fretted constantly about Ludmila and dreamed of the time we would be together again.

About three months after we arrived in Louvain I met a retired Belarusian bishop, and he introduced me to Father Robert Van-Cawelart, a Benedictine monk. During our first encounter Father Robert announced, "I am a Catholic of the Orthodox Rite. Do you consider me a heretic?" Stunned by this question, I answered, "Father Robert, heretic is a strange word to me. Belarus was home to people of many faiths, all living together. There were mixed marriages. There were few problems. You are not a heretic. You and I are as close as can be." He embraced me so tightly that I thought my ribs would break. "You know," he said, "we will be friends." And we were; ours was a wonderful, valuable friendship.

One day Father Robert asked me if my church recognized Rome as the seat of Catholic power and authority, and I said that it did. Pondering this piece of information, he suggested that we go to Rome and ask the pope for help in funding the Belarusian students. I was astonished – travelling to Rome and seeking an audience with the pope was far beyond my reach. Undaunted, Father Robert explained that he had an uncle who held an influential position in the Belgian Parliament; he might be able to help us. When I protested, Father Robert just smiled and said, "Never lose faith in what can be."

Meanwhile, another priest was helping me and the other students from Marburg obtain visas to enter Belgium. By the end of the year, our group of fifteen Belarusian refugees had found work and lodgings in Louvain. And, as promised, Father Robert had arranged a meeting with his uncle in Brussels. This gentleman had the capacity to put me at ease, and soon I found myself describing to him the problems facing Belarusian students. When he offered to set up a visit to the Vatican and an audience with the pope, I was elated. I gathered my Belarusian companions together and told them of my plan to visit Pope Pius XII. I saw the disbelief in their eyes transform into cautious hope. Two weeks later Father Robert arrived bearing the necessary documents and the confirmation of my audience with the pope, Monsignor Montini (the secretary of the Vatican

State, and later Pope Paul I), and Cardinal Tisserant, a high-ranking papal aide. It all seemed impossible, but Father Robert simply smiled and reminded me that with faith everything is possible. I knew that I was ready to do almost anything it took to finish my medical studies.

As the time of our departure drew near, Father Robert began coaching me on the proper protocol for visitors to the Vatican. He also informed me that a group of Belarusian clergy in Rome had invited me to visit them, and that they, too, would advise me on how to behave during my private audience. Many of these clerics, Father Robert confided, could not believe that a student had won an audience, especially since the pope had an unusually busy schedule in this holy year of celebrations. Finally, in early January 1950, Father Robert and I boarded a train and started our journey. As I sat quietly contemplating what the next few days would bring, Father Robert occasionally interjected with this reminder: "Never lose faith! You will succeed." His words encouraged me.

In the Holy City we were met by Vatican emissaries, who explained that I would be escorted to the Throne Room, and when the pope approached, I was to kneel. His Holiness would extend his hand, and I could decide whether or not to kiss his ring. In my awkward way, I remarked that to get a scholarship I would kiss anything! As soon as those tactless words had flown out of my mouth, I could see that I had caused offence, but Father Robert smoothed things over. We were shown to our sleeping quarters, and I had a restless night. At ten o'clock the next morning we found ourselves in Vatican City. Swiss guards checked my travel documents, and a representative of the clergy asked me what language I would like to speak when I met with the pope. Puzzled, I asked what language the pope spoke. The cleric replied that the pope would speak in the language of my choosing. After some thought, I suggested that we speak in French.

A Swiss guard addressed me in French and told me to follow him. We passed through many doors, and at each checkpoint a different person came forward to escort us to the next, until we finally arrived in the Throne Room. Standing in this magnificent room, I marvelled at the richness of the decor – there was red velvet everywhere. All around me Swiss guards stood at attention. Presently the pope arrived. He was a tall man with a pale complexion and long, delicate fingers. It struck me that if I adhered to the Catholic faith, then I could easily believe that this man was the embodiment of Christ. Everything about him assured me that I was in the presence of holiness and purity. I knelt before him and kissed his ring. He motioned for me to stand and present my problem. I had already been warned that I would have only a few minutes to speak, so I had prepared a short address, which I gave to the cardinal sitting on the pope's right. Then I began to describe the persecution we Belarusians faced and the obstacles we confronted in finishing our university studies. The pope asked me several questions, to which I responded, and then he said, "Well, Monsieur Ragula, I will pray for you, the other students, and your Christian country."

At this point I made a fortuitous diplomatic blunder. Without thinking of protocol, I said, "Your Holiness, I appreciate your prayers very much, but if you would include a scholarship, we would never forget your concern and help." I heard the cardinal gasp in disgust, and he rebuked me by saying, "How dare you ask for money when the pope was kind enough to offer his prayers!" I stood subdued and silent. I do not clearly recall much of what happened after this, but later I went to tell Father Robert about my audience, and I told him about my blunder. He laughed kindly and remarked that while my request for money had been rash, it could still have a beneficial result. Then, three weeks after our visit to Rome, his enduring faith in the possible proved itself – we received our scholarships! I thanked Montini and Tisserant for their support, but I knew that it was to Father Robert I owed the greatest debt. Without him, we Belarusian refugees in Louvain would not likely have found the means to continue our studies.

For Ludmila and me, life seemed to begin again in Belgium. We rented a house and settled into a routine of study and domestic life. In 1950 Ludmila graduated with a degree in pharmacology and later found work with several firms that dealt with the quality control of medications. A year later she gave birth to our daughter, Rahnieda, and in 1952 our son, Vitaut, came into the world.[4] Father Robert, a frequent visitor, continued to find us the material support we needed to finish our studies.

In the Catholic University medical school contact between interns and patients was limited. During lectures, which were held in large auditoriums, a patient would be presented to the class. We would take copious notes about the patient's medical history, symptoms, and treatment plan. Rarely did a student doctor have the opportunity to work with patients on the wards. I graduated in 1951 and did a locum tenens in a remote area of Belgium, quickly realizing that my lack of hands-on experience was causing discomfort for both me and my patients. For example, one day I had difficulty inserting a catheter, and I was disappointed in my clumsy efforts and disconcerted by the patient's obvious uneasiness. Over time, however, my confidence and my skills improved dramatically.

Life proceeded happily until we received news that war had broken out in Korea. Within my Belarusian community there were some who hoped that American participation in the conflict would draw world attention to the harshness of Communist rule; others wanted the Americans to destroy the Communist regime, thereby opening the door for them to return to Belarus. For many exiled Belarusians the conflict in Korea resonated with the ideological issues they had faced in their homeland during World War II – the struggle for cultural and political autonomy as well as for national identity. When Communist powers succeeded in expanding their spheres of influence, many exiled Belarusians feared reprisals and deportation. After the armistice world powers partitioned Korea into northern and southern zones of political influence. Observing this Asian conflict and its resolution, many of us were prompted to make a decision: we could either stay in Belgium or move on.

So Ludmila and I discussed our future. I recalled a book that I had read as a child in which Canada was called "the land of pine and honey." In many ways this description of Canada reminded me of Belarus. Despite some misgivings on Ludmila's part, I decided that Canada would be our new home. At the Canadian embassy I made some enquiries about our prospects, and the immigration authorities informed me that I had to have proof of employment in Canada, and that Ludmila and I would both have to pass medical exams before the immigration procedure could commence. I worked steadily to fulfill all of these requirements and wrote to sixty Canadian hospitals to apply for an internship. The College of Physicians and Surgeons of Ontario offered me a placement at St Joseph's Hospital in London, Ontario.[5] With the help of Father Robert and other Belarusian friends we prepared to leave Belgium. We would depart on 8 December 1954 from Louvain, proceed to Amsterdam by train, and board a ship for Canada.

Father Robert arranged a farewell dinner for us. Surrounded by my friends and fellow students, I had trouble keeping my emotions in check. I felt as though I were abandoning Europe, but I knew that my attachment to Belarus was as strong as ever and would remain so. On the eve of our departure my close friend Walter Nabagiez came to me and slipped an envelope into my pocket, insisting that I open it later, when we were on the ship. Once aboard I opened the envelope to discover that Walter had given us the handsome sum of $2,000! To this day, I am grateful for his generosity.[6] I stood on the deck of the ship, looking to the west and then to the east. Ludmila and the children joined me, and I told them with heartfelt conviction, "We are going to make it."

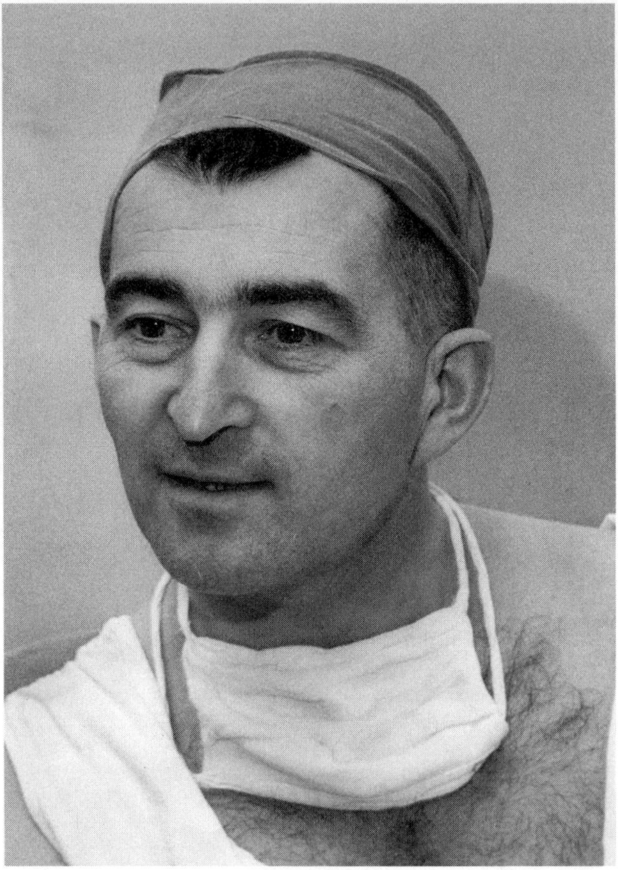

Boris as an intern at St Joseph's Hospital, c.1955

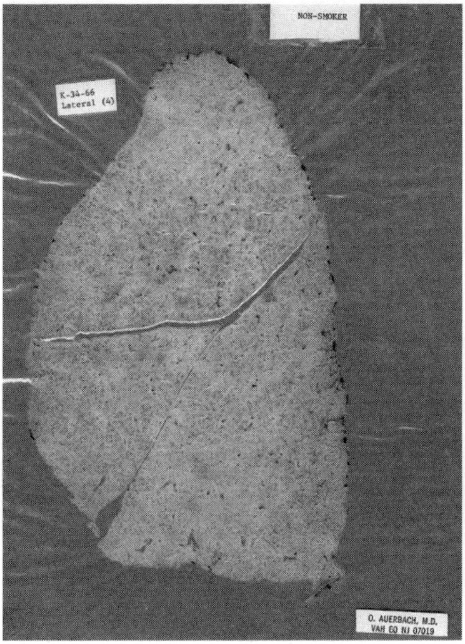

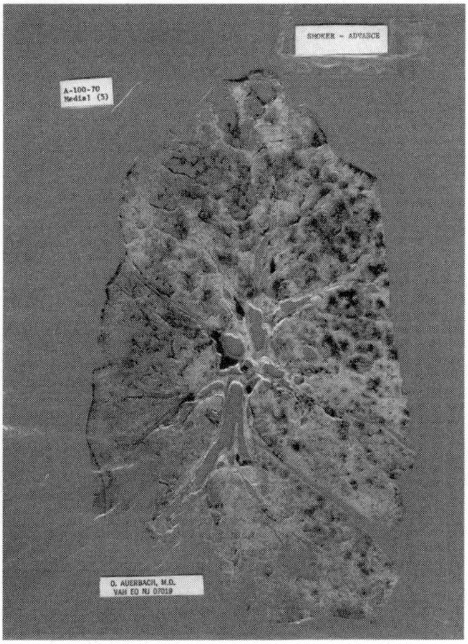

LEFT: Slide of healthy lung tissue; RIGHT: slide of diseased lung tissue. In his presentation to staff at St Joseph's Hospital, Dr Auerbach used such images to show the difference between healthy lung tissue and lung tissue damaged by smoking. Later Boris displayed this image and other materials in his waiting room

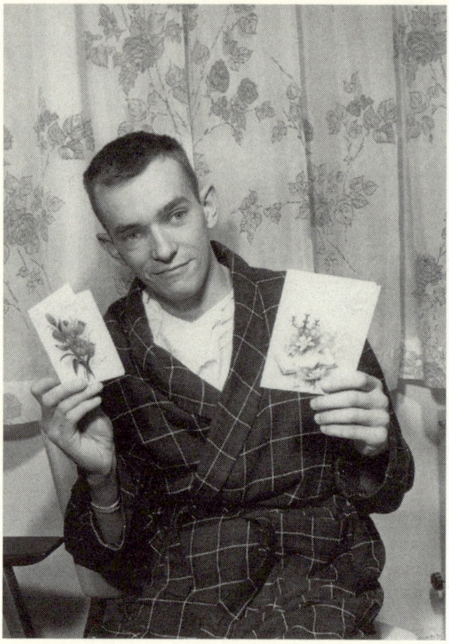

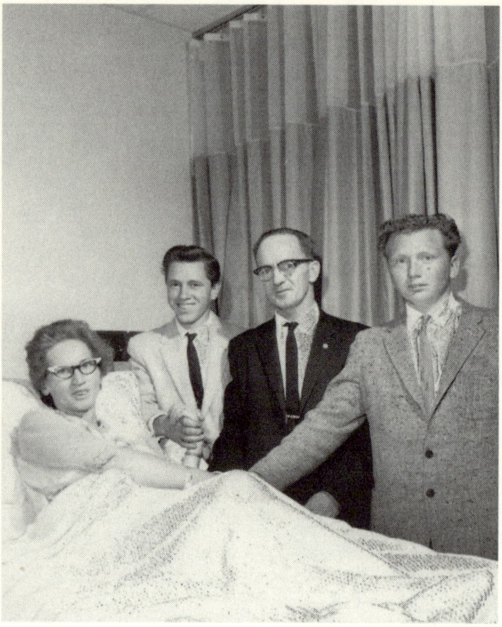

LEFT: Boris's patient Robert Bainbridge in his hospital room at St Joseph's, c.1963; RIGHT: Mrs Ackworth surrounded by her sons and husband, Easter 1963, courtesy of the J.J. Talman Regional Collection, *London Free Press* negative collection

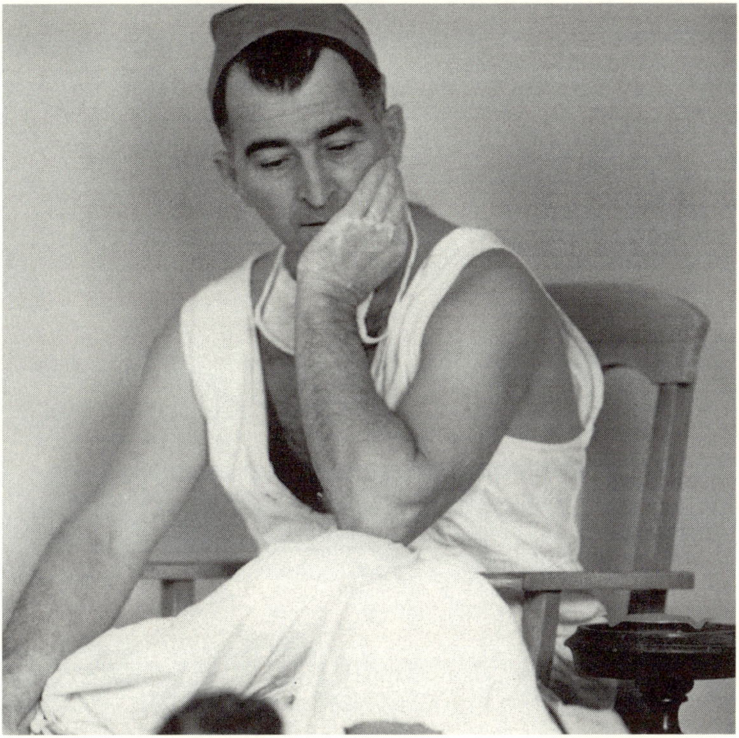

Boris, visibly exhausted, after the Bainbridge kidney transplant, 1963

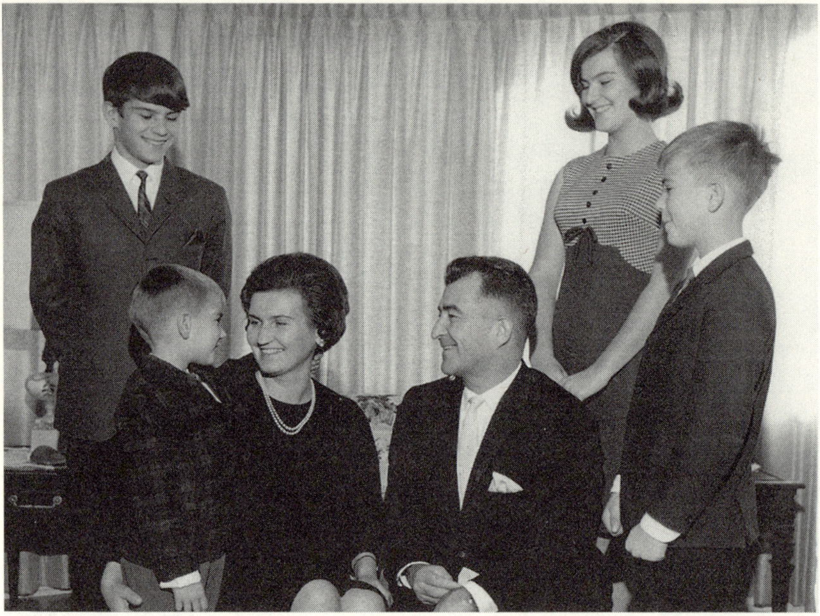

The Ragula family, c. 1964. Andrew, the youngest, stands next to his mother, Ludmila; Vitaut is in the back row, and Rahneida is behind her father, Boris; to Boris's right is Walter

6 Early Days in London, Ontario

We arrived in Toronto in December 1954. Friends had given me the address of the Belarusian Canadian Alliance, which had its offices on Dundas Street, so we hailed a taxi and made our way there. Alex Hrychuk, the president of the organization, welcomed us and helped us find temporary living quarters. Once I had settled Ludmila and the children, I set out for London. My internship was scheduled to begin on 23 December, and I wanted to see the medical director at St Joseph's Hospital without delay. It came as a great surprise to me that the director did not ask for my papers. Instead, she told me that she had all the necessary documentation and that she would find out everything she needed to know about my abilities once I had started work. I cannot recall ever showing my letters of reference from the rector of the Catholic University of Louvain or any of the other professors I worked with in Europe. "What a country!" I thought. "In Canada, people care very little for documents."

I went to the sewing room at the hospital to be fitted for my uniform, and there I met the head seamstress, Katerine. I told her that my English was poor, and she asked me if I spoke French. When I spoke to her in French, she noted that it was not my native tongue. I explained that I came from Belarus, and our conversation proceeded in Russian. This kind woman not only helped me with my uniform, but she also offered to help me find an apartment for my family. After the fitting we went together by bus to see Mrs Vondehn, who rented rooms in her rambling house on Windsor Avenue. All of Mrs Vondehn's tenants shared the main-floor kitchen. Although the apartment she had for us was small – two rooms in the attic – I signed the lease and paid a month's rent in advance. Back in Toronto, Alex introduced me to a Mr Oranski, an old friend from Belarus, who offered to drive us to London. The following day we were off. When Mr Oranski saw our new home he looked doubtful and asked, "How can you live in these cramped quarters?" Ludmila and I assured him that everything is possible if one has faith. He left us to settle in, but I am sure he had misgivings about our situation.

Ludmila looked upon the new apartment as temporary, and her immediate concern was ensuring that I could devote myself to my work without having to worry about the children's welfare. Although she could not speak much English, she managed to make herself understood. She took the children to church on Sundays, and there she established a small circle of friends and acquaintances who were always willing to help. Because of my demanding schedule at St Joseph's, I only had every other weekend free, but Ludmila did not see this as an obstacle; she refused to be isolated. She learned how to use the public transportation system. She brought the children to the hospital to visit me whenever time permitted. When we look back on these early days, we do so fondly. We may have had little in the way of material possessions, but we had something much more valuable: a shared loved and shared goals.

With some apprehension, I reported at St Joseph's on the appointed day, 23 December, and formally took up my duties as intern. In the doctors' lounge I met my colleagues. Dr Bill Keel was the only English-speaking intern in the hospital; the rest of the group was comprised of two Russians, a Romanian, a German, a Yugoslav, a Pole, and an East Indian (the only woman). Most of the interns had already been working at the hospital for two or three years, and many of them were struggling to learn English. Our lounge conversations would have seemed quite comical to outsiders. Relying on our imaginations, some animated gestures, and a smattering of our native languages, we somehow communicated very well. We were bound together by the fact that we were all working hard to build successful careers as Canadian doctors. At St Joseph's interns were expected to cover a medical ward with 450 beds, work in the emergency department, scrub for the operating theatre, and deliver babies. We spent three days on shift and two days off. One of my early successes, which I owed to a patient, involved compiling a medical history. The patient in question, a high school teacher, related to me in great detail his past illnesses, symptoms, and treatments, but when I conducted a physical examination I found him to be in good general health except for a hernia, which had to be repaired surgically. I was able to use this sample medical history as a model throughout my first year as an intern, and it helped me to gain confidence in my abilities.

Early in my internship I learned that I would have to pass an examination to attain enabling certification. Once I had leapt this academic hurdle I would be eligible to write the Ontario Medical Council examinations, provided that I had also completed at least one year of my internship program. The enabling certification examinations covered several topics: biochemistry, pathology, physiology, and English. I signed up for the examinations set for February 1955 against the advice of my fellow interns – a number of them had written the examinations and failed for a variety of reasons. Many had had difficulty with the English aspect of the exams, but I knew that there were some English-language courses available that could be accommodated to a busy intern's schedule, and I resolved to study hard to improve my fragmented English as quickly as possible. Another deterrent, which had stopped many of my colleagues from taking the examinations, was the fifty-dollar administration fee (a large sum of money for an intern on a meagre stipend) plus the cost of travel to the examination centre in Toronto. Somehow I would scrape the money together. Since I had graduated from medical school quite recently, I reasoned that I should put my knowledge to the test while it was still fresh. However, my decision to take the exams so soon turned my life into something of a nightmare. Every waking minute I spent working and studying. Without Ludmila's help I doubt that I would have succeeded. Despite the tension we were under, we were too busy to argue or squabble. All our energies were focused on studying and maintaining the family.

While intensive study had the effect of improving my English, and while it became apparent that my knowledge of other languages (including Latin) helped as well, I started to have serious doubts about my level of preparedness as the weeks flew by. I had some confidence in my knowledge of anatomy and physiology, but many concepts in biochemistry had changed since 1946, and I had to admit that my spoken and written English were still weak. Nevertheless, before I knew it I was in Toronto checking into a hotel near the examination centre. Anatomy came first. As I was unfamiliar with many of the English anatomy terms, I decided to use their Latin equivalents. This proved to be a good strategy, because Latin was still listed as the language of origin for anatomy, so my answers were accepted. Aside from this, I remember little of the first day of the examinations except that it thoroughly exhausted me. Biochemistry was the second scheduled exam. In order to avoid mistakes I decided to write everything in chemical formulae. During the oral portion the examiner had no option but to discuss the answers in the same format. At one point he noted that I had made an error in the lengthy formula for coenzyme A. Without missing a beat I gave him the specific reference and the correct answer. He peered at me over his spectacles and asked me to write another chemical formula. Again I took pen and paper, but before I had finished the exercise he exclaimed, "You make me sick!" At this point I became rather flustered and worried because I had taken him literally. Nonplussed, the examiner explained that he was not in fact ill, and he added that he had never before received a paper written entirely in chemical formulae. He was impressed with my efforts.

My marks on the technical examinations exceeded 90 per cent, on average. However, I struggled and faltered during the English-proficiency test. Although the examiner tried her best to make me feel less anxious, I knew that I had performed dismally. As I prepared to leave the examination room, this kind woman told me that my English was remarkable given my short time in Canada, and she was confident that I would master the language by the time I faced the licensing board. Troubled and uncertain about the outcome, I returned to London to await the examination results. When I arrived home Ludmila took one look at my face and then embraced me saying that she "knew" I had passed. Swayed by her loving confidence, I danced with her around our small apartment. It was a dance of hope.

Rather than brood while awaiting my results, I threw myself into my work on the wards. One day a senior staff member in gynecology asked me to write a medical history for a patient booked for a hysterectomy. The doctor's diagnosis was that she had a mass in her uterus. As luck would have it, the patient was Ukrainian and spoke Russian. She told me that she was thirty-nine years old and that her last period had occurred approximately three months earlier. After recording this information, I examined her and told her that I did not think she needed surgery. In fact, congratulations were in order – she was about three months pregnant! She looked askance, but I promised her that I would confer with the specialist who had told her she required a hysterectomy to ensure that my diagnosis was correct. I explained all of this to the head nurse, who insisted that I take the matter up with the presiding surgeon, so I called him and explained in my broken English that in my opinion the patient was pregnant, and I was recommending that the hysterectomy be postponed until further tests could be done. He nearly ruptured my eardrum when he started yelling into the phone that I should keep my opinions to myself, do my duty as an intern, and stop questioning "qualified" staff. Then he slammed down the receiver.

Although shaken by this response, I was guided by my conscience. I went back to the patient and told her that the only way for her to avoid surgery was to refuse to sign the consent form. She assured me that although she thought she was a bit old to be having a child, she did not want to end the pregnancy. When the surgeon learned that his patient had refused to sign the consent form he severed all professional associations with me. About six months later the patient, whose name was Nadia, delivered a healthy baby boy, and when I eventually opened my own practice she sought me out and asked me to be her family physician. Ludmila met Nadia at church soon after her child was born. Nadia put the cherub in Ludmila's arms and exclaimed, "Without your husband I would not have this child!" Ludmila replied, "I think your husband had more to do with this baby than Boris did!" When the baby, whom Nadia affectionately nicknamed "the tumour," came in for his regular check-ups, I felt elated and somehow blessed that another child had come into this world. Aside from this incident I had very few conflicts with senior or supervising staff during my years as an intern. The staff at St Joseph's consistently demonstrated excellence in their work; this isolated case of misdiagnosis serves only as a reminder that doctors are human and fallible. We make mistakes but, with the support of our colleagues and staff, we rarely jeopardize our patients' well-being.

I was taking a break in the doctors' lounge one day when the mail boy handed me a letter from the Ontario College of Physicians and Surgeons. My colleagues watched as I opened it, knowing, as I did, that it contained my examination results. They had heard me express my opinion about the structure and intent of examinations; I thought that regulated testing was geared towards the average student, not the genius. After I had read the letter I took a deep breath and threw it on the coffee table. "Well, Boris, what is the news?" asked my friends. "Read it yourselves," I said quietly. "I passed." We had little time for celebrating, but I do remember feeling tremendously relieved.

Work at the hospital continued at a steady pace. I recall it as a challenging time, one of observation and learning. With the enabling examinations behind me, I applied for a residency in medicine with the option to resign depending on the results of my final licensing board examinations. I turned down a residency in surgery that many of my colleagues coveted. As a result, some staff began to regard me as someone who went against the standard. They did not understand that my goal as a medical doctor was to reach out to patients in the same way my father had. Perhaps it was a philosophy and an approach to medicine born of eastern European culture and values. These days the family physician plays a much more important role in health care, but early in my career I noted that many young interns and doctors turned to specialization, which offered a status and a medical focus that a general family practice could not provide.

So, for the duration of my internship, I worked hard at the hospital, studied for my final examinations, and tried to find time to spend with my growing family. I wrote the exams, and in June 1956 the College of Physicians and Surgeons informed me that I had passed. I now had my license to practise independently in the province of Ontario. I find it difficult even now to express my feelings about this in words. Of course, I felt as though I had cast off a heavy burden of uncertainty, but I was still anxious and insecure. However, when I told Ludmila that I had decided to continue working at St Joseph's and open a private practice in London, she bolstered my confidence in the idea that we could build a future for ourselves; we could put the concentration camps, the food shortages, and all the suffering behind us. Ludmila looked after our young brood, and she also managed to hold down a part-time job at a local pharmacy; after our youngest son, Walter, arrived she became a stay-at-home mother.

With a loan of $3,000 from my cousin Michael Ragula, who lived in New York City, I made a down payment on 756 Adelaide Street in London.[1] On the ground floor of the house were an office, a reception area, and examination rooms. The living room became my waiting room. Ludmila used the kitchen for family meals, and we lived in the three bedrooms on the second floor. Once we had organized the office and living spaces, I hung my shingle at the front of the house and waited for patients.

Until I could hire a receptionist, Ludmila agreed to fill in. It was August 1956, and she had just given birth to our third child, Walter. It was quite a juggling act for her, but she managed it, and we still chuckle at the memory of some of the encounters she had with patients in those early days. On one occasion a new patient phoned for an appointment, and, of course, Ludmila answered in English. At the other end of the line she heard an angry voice complain in Ukrainian to someone else that he had some idiot on the phone who could not speak his language. Unperturbed, Ludmila addressed the caller in Ukrainian and made the appointment. It struck us both as somewhat comical that a person living in Canada expected service in his native tongue. A few weeks later I hired Betty, a co-worker of Ludmila's when she worked in a local pharmacy, as my receptionist. Relieved of her office duties, Ludmila applied herself to keeping our active children occupied while I held office hours. It became apparent to both of us that the family and my practice could not flourish under one roof, so two years later, in May 1958, we bought a house just north of Windermere Drive, and there we have lived ever since.

My Adelaide Street practice grew steadily. Unlike my colleagues at St Joseph's, I spoke a number of European languages, and this helped to break down barriers for new Canadians trying to assimilate into North American life. These immigrants approached me not only for their medical needs, but also for help with translation and job hunting. Another reason that my practice prospered was that I adhered to a personal philosophy of family medicine: patients always took precedence. I made house calls, I took patients with or without appointments, and I opened my door to anyone in need at any time. Of course, this commitment took its toll on my family life, but Ludmila never complained. She dedicated herself to the children with the same energy and enthusiasm that I gave to my patients. After many months of taking payment for my services in the form of eggs, cabbage rolls, and other goods, I finally earned my first dollar as a physician. The pride that I took in earning this money was related to a concept of value that derived from being denied the opportunity to pursue personal goals by a repressive Communist regime. Holding the money in my hands, I vowed from then on to donate a portion of my earnings to the causes of fighting Communism and aiding those trapped behind the Iron Curtain.

While living in Germany and Belgium during the post-war years I had played an active role in Belarusian student organizations, including serving as president of the Belarusian Student Council of Western Europe. I relinquished this post in 1952, but I maintained contact with the organization and its membership. In Canada I became a member of the Belarusian Canadian Alliance and stood as president of the organization in 1963 and again in 1965. Ten years later I would become president of the Belarusian Coordinating Committee, which had its headquarters in Toronto. I also worked with the Belarusian Democratic Council in Exile. Perhaps to those who have never suffered degradation or experienced the suppression of their ethnic or basic human rights my allegiance to Belarusian groups seems like a denial of my new Canadian citizenship, but that impression is false. In fact, the freedom I enjoyed as a new Canadian and the material success I had been able to achieve in Canada allowed me to extend aid to those living in the dark shadow cast by totalitarian regimes.

In my practice I met people from all walks of life who understood the true value of life and living. I would like to pay tribute here to one such person – Mrs Ackworth, a forty-four-year-old grandmother – who demonstrated not only courage but also an admirable selflessness. Since 1956 I had been treating a young man named Robert Bainbridge for glomerulonephritis, a disease in which small, fibre-like units in the kidney become inflamed and unable to perform their normal function of filtering waste products from the blood. Robert's condition gradually worsened, and by 1963 his consulting doctors and surgeons had come to believe that a kidney transplant was Robert's only chance for survival. One day I was on the phone discussing Robert's case with urologist Dr Lionel Reese when Mrs Ackworth, in the waiting room, chanced to overhear part of our conversation. As soon as I hung up the phone, she came into my office and offered to donate one of her kidneys to Robert. I was astounded! I explained to her that two members of Robert's family and his girlfriend had already offered to be donors, but they did not meet the medical requirements. Undeterred, Mrs Ackworth insisted that she be tested. I laid out the risks involved and advised her to go home and discuss it with her husband. Mrs Ackworth persisted, we ran a battery of tests, and she proved to be a suitable donor. When I asked her why she felt compelled to make such a sacrifice for a complete stranger, she said, "I want to live as long as I can. I'm sure Robert does, too. If you see someone drowning you don't stand and watch. You jump in and help." I replied softly, "Mrs Ackworth, you are going to jump quite a long way."

Robert and Mrs Ackworth met for the first time as they were being wheeled into the operating theatre. She told me afterwards that when she saw Robert, who was only twenty-one, lying there so pale and weak, she thought of her robust sons and knew she was doing the right thing. The local and regional newspapers carried reports about this remarkable woman in which they described in detail the ordeal of the then-controversial organ transplant. This was only the second kidney transplant that had ever been performed in London. Officials at St Joseph's, with the consent of the families of the donor and the recipient, invited *London Free Press* reporter Del Bell and photographer Jeanne Graham to observe and record the five-hour operation. Dr Vincent Callaghan, chief of surgery at St Joseph's, Dr Reese, and Dr S.E. Carroll, a cardiovascular surgeon, performed the procedures; I assisted Reese and Carroll in the operating theatre. After it was all over, the exhausted Reese and Carroll sat for a few minutes in the staff lounge talking to reporters. Everything went well, they said, but they also warned that every day would be a milestone. The possibility of infection and the body's natural tendency to reject foreign matter were unquestionably the most crucial factors.[2]

Robert's struggle to live ended almost two months after the transplant. Mrs Ackworth had visited him in the hospital during the post-surgery recovery period, and when she heard that he had died she said, "He was a fine young man – every mother's dream of a good son." I think that Robert summed it up best on his way into the operating theatre, when he held out his hand to Mrs Ackworth and whispered, "Thank you."

Very early in my practice I became involved with preventative medicine. My interest in this area was sparked in the spring of 1959, when a female patient of about forty came to me complaining of lower-back pain. Her name was Olga. I took her medical history and gave her a physical examination, but I could not make a diagnosis. I explained to her that her pain could be due to some disorder of the bowel or reproductive organs. Olga reluctantly gave me permission to proceed with a pelvic examination, and I noted an unusual bloody discharge as well as erosions around the cervix. I suspected a connection between these observed abnormalities and the pain she was experiencing. When I suggested that a cervical biopsy and a dilation and curettage (D and C) would help me determine the root problem, she accused me of trying to use these tests for financial gain.[3] Visibly upset, she refused to undergo further testing and left my office. A few weeks later she returned to inform me that she had seen a gynecologist, and he had told her that everything was fine. I knew that something had been overlooked, so after she left I called the gynecologist and requested that he proceed with a biopsy since I had a strong suspicion of cervical cancer. He became indignant and insisted that I lacked an understanding of his particular field of expertise. I even went so far as to speak with Olga's husband, who commiserated with me but maintained that his wife was a stubborn woman who refused to believe that she had anything seriously the matter with her, especially cancer. Although I had grave concerns, there was nothing more that I could do for this patient without her consent.

Some months later I saw Olga at the hospital. She was under the care of another doctor, a surgeon, who informed me that she was in labour, but she had serious complications and would require a surgical delivery. The surgeon was very concerned because a distraught Olga had claimed that she was going to sue me. I examined her charts and discovered that her problems were, as I had suspected months ago, due to cervical cancer, which was by now advanced. My heart sank, for I knew that this could have been prevented. Nonetheless, I went to see Olga in her room, and she hurled insults and threats at me. I let her scream and cry because I felt that she needed some emotional release. When she had settled down a bit, I sat by her bed and tried to comfort her. She turned her tear-stained face to me and said, "Doctor, this is all my fault."

My experience with Olga inspired me to research ways in which early diagnosis of cervical cancer could be introduced into the regime of regular physical examinations for women. I contacted Dr J. Walters, head of gynecology and obstetrics at St Joseph's. In 1959 Walters had founded London's first cancer cytology laboratory. In its first year his clinic performed 800 Pap smears on healthy women in order to identify abnormal cell growth, which could indicate cancer of the cervix.[4] In 1960, after consulting with Dr Walters, I started what might be termed an independent study: I had Pap smears done on all my female patients between the ages of twenty and sixty. Over a seven-year period my small study indicated that approximately one woman in one hundred had positive cells associated with carcinoma of the cervix. I asked Dr Walters to conduct an objective review of my results; he did this for me, and he gave me his support. In 1967 he encouraged me to present a paper on my findings at the third congress of the American Cancer Cytology Society, to be held in New York City in May. I went to New York and stood at the podium before an audience of renowned medical men and women, feeling out of my element because as a general practitioner I had little standing in the hierarchy of the medical profession. Nonetheless, the audience demonstrated a remarkable degree of interest and enthusiasm for my initiative. And, as a further endorsement, the *Journal of American Cancer Cytology* published a paper I wrote on the subject the following year.[5]

Back in London Dr Walters and I worked together to set up an outpatient clinic for women between the ages of eighteen and sixty-five. Determined to bring this important information to the public, I spoke at schools and factories – anywhere I could find an audience interested in preventative medicine. All of the hard work I was pouring into my private practice and my research left me exhausted and weak. In 1968, during our annual family vacation, I suffered what was eventually diagnosed as a relapse of the tuberculosis I had acquired as a prisoner in the Soviet Union. Years before, my grandmother had performed a medical miracle by nursing me back to health with good food, sunshine, fresh air, and exercise, and the disease had gone into remission, lying dormant until years later, when my resistance was low. I had blood in my urine and pain in my kidney, and these symptoms compelled me to seek medical advice. I went to see Dr Lionel Reese, who sent me to the hospital for tests and observation. Before TB was identified as the root cause of my problems, Reese spoke candidly with Ludmila, telling her that I had a kidney infection that could indicate cancer. He explained to my badly frightened wife that further tests were needed. Months later Ludmila confided to me that she had left Reese's office in a daze, found the car in the hospital parking lot, and driven around aimlessly for an hour. Suddenly aware that she was north of the city limits, she turned around and headed home to find solace in prayer and the children. Once Reese had diagnosed TB, I agreed to follow his advice and take a six-month leave of absence. I arranged for a young doctor to take over my practice, but I only agreed to short periods of hospitalization. With Ludmila's care and practical assistance, I was determined to regain my health.

During one hospital stint I asked Reese to remove my infected kidney so I could resume my normal activities, but he convinced me that such a drastic measure was unnecessary. A new antibiotic drug had been discovered, and this medication, coupled with Ludmila's constant attention, gradually brought the infection under control. I was a reluctant and at times uncooperative patient. Because I refused to have a nurse disrupt our household, Ludmila had to learn how to administer my daily injections of antibiotics. As I was unaccustomed to being idle, I used the time to study for examinations that would qualify me to lecture at the faculty of medicine at the University of Western Ontario. When the house felt too cramped, I would go to the backyard and shovel out a cozy hollow in the deep snow. There, shielded from the wind, I would make myself comfortable and bask in the early-winter sunshine as I followed my self-imposed study regime. Now, when the family gathers for a visit, we sometimes reminisce about those difficult months when Papa was not in his office. I do not know where Ludmila found the strength to carry on during this trying time – she cared for me, did the housework, and took the children to dance lessons, swimming, and other sporting activities. She ran the household efficiently and never lost faith. Ludmila is, and always has been, my most precious helpmate, friend, and lover. When I felt well enough I insisted on going to the local arena to watch my son play hockey. Reese objected strenuously, insisting that by breathing the damp, cold arena air I was jeopardizing my recovery. Rather than argue, Ludmila just ensured that I was well bundled up and sent me on my way.

By the spring of 1969 I had regained my health, and I eagerly plunged back into my work. My first priority was to rebuild my private practice. Many of my patients did not have confidence in the young doctor who had replaced me. Perhaps he was overwhelmed by the task or ill-equipped to give patients as much time and personal attention as I had. In any case, many patients had gone elsewhere, but they slowly came back to my practice and my professional life returned to normal. By "normal," however, I do not mean to imply stagnant. My commitment to serve my community and to pursue causes and programs that I deeply believed in was renewed. In the early 1970s I passed the qualifying examinations and attained certification from the College of Family Physicians. This allowed me to take medical students into my practice to fulfill their locum requirements. I also made time to explore new areas of preventive medicine. Although these activities secured me a place of prominence in the medical community, I felt that I had just begun my work.

7 Community Service Far and Wide

Much of my involvement with preventative medicine programs came about through my interactions with patients in my practice. One day I attended a female patient who was recovering from a heart attack. Nursing staff had just removed her from an oxygen tent, and I stood by her hospital bed anxious to know how she was feeling. I was a smoker at the time, and I lit up as I spoke with her. She sat up and watched me inhale the tobacco smoke, and then she asked me for a cigarette. Outraged, I started to berate the woman for attempting to smoke when she knew that she had heart disease, failing to see my own hypocrisy in lecturing on the evils of tobacco while holding a burning cigarette. The patient gave me a puzzled look and then asked me not to smoke in front of her. If she could find the will-power to quit smoking, she insisted, then I could too, and I should not presume to criticize her for smoking if I was going to continue to light up. Her words hit home, and at 10:15 a.m. on 3 May 1957 I threw my cigarettes away. That woman taught me a valuable lesson and inadvertently propelled me into another community program, one that many of my colleagues did not initially endorse.

In the late 1950s and early 1960s it was permissible to smoke in all medical institutions and offices. A pungent haze of tobacco smoke clouded most doctors' waiting rooms and offices, as well as hospital wards and lounges. Cigarette smoking was socially and culturally acceptable. When I began to advocate the elimination of smoking in medical facilities, many prominent physicians protested vehemently – they strongly believed that this would infringe upon their personal freedom. Some were profoundly insulted because they thought that my push to ensure a smoke-free medical environment implied that they had neglected the welfare of their patients. I knew that I was facing an uphill battle, so I decided to proceed on two fronts. First, I would disseminate scientific evidence of the link between smoking and poor health with the goal of separating the intellectual smoker from the emotional one. Second, I would approach authorities of public institutions, like the hospitals, and try to convince them to eliminate, or at least limit, patients' exposure to tobacco smoke.

After doing some research I contacted Dr Oscar Auerbach of New Jersey, who had conducted a study to evaluate the effects of tobacco smoke. Early in his project, which he had launched in 1954, he exposed twenty-four dogs to tobacco smoke. He had attached smoking machines to their throats, and while a few resisted this exposure, the majority of the subject dogs were soon hooked, much like human smokers. Auerbach then took samples of the dogs' saliva to test for the presence of premalignant cells. He recorded his results and then separated the dogs with premalignant cells into two groups: one would become smoke-free; the other would continue to be exposed to tobacco smoke. The dogs in the second group developed cancerous cells within eight months, while the dogs in the first group regained their health and showed no signs of malignancy.[1] Although Auerbach's early tests were not given much support by the American and Canadian Medical Associations, I thought that his findings were worth sharing with my colleagues and the general public.

I invited Dr Auerbach to come to London in September 1971 as my guest, and I arranged for him to present his research to a gathering of medical professionals at St Joseph's Hospital. He showed slides and films that dramatically illustrated what smoking does to healthy lung tissue. When interviewed by a local reporter, Auerbach stated that "there is no question that one doctor smoking cigarettes is worse than 5,000 lay people smoking." In other words, as informed professionals, physicians had a duty to set a good example.[2]

Resistance to my anti-smoking position was evident everywhere. One of my patients, a male high school teacher with a three-pack-a-day habit, adamantly rejected my warnings. During a regular physical examination I took a saliva sample from him, and the test results indicated the presence of precancerous cells. I did my best to convince him to stop smoking, but he listened with mounting anger and spat out, "I am not a dog." He found another family physician. Three years later I encountered him at St Joseph's. He had developed full-blown lung cancer. In a matter of months, despite surgery and treatment, he died an agonizing death. Then one evening a ward nurse called me to the hospital because one of my patients had developed chest pains. When I arrived on the four-bed ward I surveyed the situation. The patients in the other three beds were smoking, and their visitors were also puffing away. There was no doubt in my mind that second-hand smoke was contributing to my patient's distress. Calling the nursing sister to the ward, I insisted that she clear the area of cigarette smokers. She hesitated, and I threatened to call the *London Free Press* and report her negligence. "Don't test me, sister," I warned. "I will make this call if you do not exercise your authority and clear this ward. Your negligence is killing my patient." Yes, these were strong words, but I meant them, and they had the desired effect. Soon after this incident the hospital's medical advisory committee implemented a policy prohibiting visitors from smoking on the wards, but it stopped short of imposing a total ban on smoking in the hospital.

I realized from the outset that my goal of mounting a fully sanctioned and medically endorsed anti-smoking campaign would not be easily achieved. During my tenure as president of the London and District Academy of Medicine I obtained the backing of the general council of the Ontario Medical Association (OMA) for my campaign.[3] In September 1974 the OMA instructed its committee on public health to "view with alarm the lack of response of the public to the multiple dangers of smoking." Interviewed by the local press, I commented that "it was no use banning smoking in patient areas by the public if doctors continued to smoke."[4] With my encouragement, the Academy of Medicine started to organize an anti-smoking campaign in co-operation with local boards of education. We also formulated a general plan to take our message to people where they lived and worked.

Frequently I observed that every positive achievement we saw in our public health initiative was met with persuasive negative arguments, even from within the ranks of committed non-smokers. In January 1977 the *London Free Press* carried an article that clearly outlined the battle still to be fought. According to Gar Mahood, director of the Non-smokers' Rights Association, the Ontario Ministry of Health's guidelines for non-smoking areas in public places were "misleading and unacceptable and cannot work." Mahood called for legislation instead of the voluntary guidelines, which simply requested that "public places such as hospitals, cinemas, restaurants and food and department stores set up non-smoking areas." He maintained that enforcing "legislation against smoking in public areas would be difficult or impossible" and that the government's failure to curb tobacco advertising would undermine the anti-smoking campaign's chances for success.[5] In many ways Mahood's words were prophetic. It would take almost thirty years for the ministry to impose limitations on tobacco advertising. At the municipal level anti-smoking campaigns have only recently been given legal bite with bylaws governing smoking in public places. When I look back on my involvement with anti-smoking groups I realize that I was in good company. Through various agencies and organizations, thousands of us worked, and continue to work, diligently to make the public aware of the dangers of smoking. Perhaps in the future tobacco use will be universally scorned and reviled as self-destructive behaviour.

I often made time to debate political and social issues as well. I submitted briefs, letters, and articles to government agencies in which I voiced my opinions and observations on a wide array of subjects, including the Belarusian Canadian Alliance, biculturalism and bilingualism, and the prominent role the family physician can play in effecting social change. By 1970 I considered myself an "average Canadian" with a stake in the future of this promising country. Perhaps out of a sense of adventure, or curiosity, or both, I offered my services to the federal government to work in the Northwest Territories. The response was swift: government authorities sent me to Inuvik for the month of August. To reach the town, which had been established in 1961 as part of Prime Minister John Diefenbaker's "vision of the north," I flew to Edmonton and transferred to a government plane, which soared over the sixtieth parallel. Lush farmlands disappeared and were replaced by a landscape of sparse vegetation and a scattering of small settlements. The panorama below me – the breathtaking Mackenzie River delta, the towns of Hay River, Yellowknife, and Norman Wells – had an indelible impact on my senses.

At this time discoveries of large oil reserves in Alaska and the Canadian Arctic were provoking a great deal of interest in the North. This interest, in turn, prompted renewed concerns about the social and economic problems of northern Aboriginal populations. I had read many articles accusing the federal government of neglecting the health and welfare of these people, but during my short stay in Inuvik I formed an entirely different point of view. I came to believe that the average Native northerner had better access to medical care than someone living in densely populated southwestern Ontario. Inuvik General Hospital had one hundred beds, with an average occupancy rate of between fifty-one and eighty patients. These patients came from isolated settlements such as Aklavik, Fort McPherson, Fort Good Hope, and Sachs Harbour. Doctors and nurses flew to these settlements on a monthly basis to offer general clinics that included prenatal assessment, well-baby examinations, and inoculations. If the local nurse had a seriously ill patient and required assistance, she would contact Inuvik General by radio and confer with the doctor on duty. Should they determine that specialized care was necessary, the patient would be air-lifted to Inuvik, usually within four to six hours of the radio consultation.

Sometimes doctors would travel to the outpost settlements to give on-site treatment. The summer I was in the North a prospector broke his back at Banks Island, five hundred miles from Inuvik. A doctor, accompanied by a nurse, flew to the settlement to evaluate the man's condition, and after he had done so he ordered another plane to transport the patient to Vancouver for neurological treatment. Many members of the Native community shunned such services for a variety of reasons. For one thing they remembered the devastating tuberculosis outbreak of the 1940s, after which few of the patients sent south by the medical authorities for specialized treatment returned home.

I did not spend all of my time in the North working. Early in my visit I was invited to attend a banquet in honour of the governor general of Canada, the Right Honourable D. Roland Michener. Michener was an avid sportsman and athlete who exercised daily. During a lull in the festivities he asked if anyone would care to go jogging with him the next morning. I gladly volunteered, and we arranged to meet at 7 a.m. When I arrived at his quarters his attendants asked me to wait – Mr Michener was still asleep. The attendants scurried off to perform their official duties, and I knocked on Michener's door. He answered my knock looking a bit tousled, but he was not in the least concerned about my breach of protocol. We enjoyed an instant rapport. Flanked by his bodyguards, we set off on that crisp, clear Inuvik morning. Although Michener was twenty years my senior, I found myself working hard to keep pace; furthermore, the governor general liked to converse while jogging, which I found somewhat taxing. Michener asked me about my background and my thoughts on the state of Canadian society. One of his questions concerned my position on the monarchy. I took my time formulating an appropriate answer, but then I decided that frankness, rather than obsequiousness, was the best approach. "Your Excellency," I replied, "I come from a European background and so I am not familiar with the Canadian and British structures of monarchy. In my country, monarchs are native-born. However, if you were the monarch of Canada, I would freely give my allegiance to the Canadian monarchy." Michener looked at me and then broke out in a wide smile. "Dr Ragula," he said, "I understand your feelings."

I had no inkling that Michener would remember our brief encounter. However, a year later, when Michener opened the Stratford Festival, he happened to meet a patient of mine named Richard Moore. It somehow came up in their conversation that Moore was one of my patients, and Michener asked him why Dr Ragula had not come to the festival. Imagine my reaction! This public figure, who met thousands of people while performing his duties, had remembered me, an obscure family physician. One of my prized possessions is a photograph of the two of us jogging, which the governor general sent to me in 1972. The inscription reads, "To Dr Boris Ragula, with fond regards from your friend Roland Michener."

Inuvik General arranged for me to spend two days working in the Aklavik clinic. Located on the west shore of the Peel Channel in the Mackenzie delta, Aklavik had a population of about eight hundred. Most were Aboriginal, but I also met a few white people employed by power installations, trading posts, the airport, the churches, and the RCMP. To my eyes the ridges of the Richardson Mountains, the site of many battles between warring indigenous tribes, added a secular beauty to Aklavik. The nursing station in this small community was well equipped. On the ground floor I found the general reception area, a large room housing an X-ray machine, facilities for processing and storing medical supplies, and examination cubicles. On the second floor was another examining room with equipment for performing minor surgery, a dispensary, and four hospital beds. Supervising staff reserved one bed for obstetrics and one for contagious diseases. I also noted the isolation wards and two hospital rooms used to treat patients suffering from ailments such as pneumonia or heart problems. Here patients could be comfortable while receiving treatment requiring a short hospital stay. When I arrived at the Aklavik clinic there was only one patient in residence, and she was recovering from childbirth. I met with the clinic nurse, and she outlined her daily routine for me, showing me how she conducted her morning clinics and planned her afternoon house calls. The local population considered the nursing station and clinic a community meeting place, and I witnessed many residents seeking advice on issues unrelated to medical problems. It was clear to me that settlement nurses played a vital role in northern communities by reaching out to the locals as both professionals and friends.

During a scheduled house call I had the opportunity to visit a home for the elderly. Although the exterior of the building was dreary and unimpressive, inside the place was warm and pleasant. There was a large living room furnished with soft chairs and sofas; a sparkling, well-organized kitchen; and twelve bedrooms, each with a bed, a chair or sofa, a small table, and a closet for storing personal belongings. While making the rounds I met an old prospector who had originally come from England. Staff told me that he had kept his bags packed for the past twenty-five years because he believed that he would soon be returning to his homeland. He sat happily puffing on his pipe and dreaming of verdant England.

I discovered that in the Northwest Territories a house call could be quite an adventure. Accompanied by another doctor and a nurse, I flew in a Cessna four-seater to the settlement of Paulatuk. The view from the air was magnificent – an immense treeless vista of lakes and rivers. I was enthralled by the beauty of this wild terrain as I gazed down at the Anderson River, with its high banks on one side and deep canyons on the other. The pilot pointed out several herds of caribou and the occasional moose. Once we passed over the Horton River, Paulatuk came into sight. On our descent brilliant sunlight illuminated the land below, and I felt as though I were being welcomed into an ethereal world.

Paulatuk consisted of nine prefabricated cottage-style homes and a church. The nursing station was a trailer. We began to receive our patients, and I was struck by the fact that not one of the young children I examined cried or even showed any fear. They were quiet, watchful, and curious. A three-year-old girl, perhaps misled by my deep suntan, pointed at me and said questioningly to her mother, "Tanaluk," which means "white man." I teased her a little, putting my tanned arm close to hers, and she repeated insistently "Tanaluk!" When I asked her who she was, she replied "Inuit" – "person" or "human being." Her answer gave me a lot to think about. At the end of the day I sought out an Aboriginal elder because I wanted to learn something of their history and culture. I told him about my encounter with the little girl and asked him the meaning of "Inuit." He looked at me carefully before he replied. "In a way," he said, "the Inuit are different from the Tanaluk. We do not fight, we do not kill anyone, and we do not take another's land. We are a peaceful people. We like one another. Maybe that is why we consider ourselves Inuit – human beings. Tanaluk are not like us." Here in this seemingly barren land, among unsophisticated people, I had rediscovered the true meaning of humanity. Alone, with time to mull over all that I had seen and heard, I recalled the degradation and the terror to which the Red Army and the Nazis had subjected innocent people. The Inuit view of humanity made so much more sense than the view of "civilized" white people.

The Inuit belief system was characterized by a rare purity, but I was alarmed to observe signs of the erosion of their social and cultural structures. Among the older clinic patients tuberculosis continued to be a serious problem. Medical files also disclosed that venereal disease was widespread in the community. Some authorities attributed this to the influx of transient workers, businesspeople, and travellers who exploited the Aboriginals for their own pleasure. Alcohol abuse was another serious threat – many teenagers and young adults seemed to think that every bottle should be emptied. I asked a young female patient why she used alcohol, and she replied that life was boring and the buzz from alcohol provided a temporary escape. I later realized that I had witnessed the beginnings of the devastating changes that would wreak havoc among the Inuit and other Aboriginal peoples. With every incursion by an oil company or some other development enterprise, these people lost traditional lands, and this in turn weakened their local economies and their cultural and community structures. Yet, despite these problems, I shall always remember my brief sojourn in Canada's North as a unique adventure.

Back in London, I continued to work with other medical practitioners and patients to improve and expand programs dealing with a wide assortment of health-related topics. Through my association with the London Health Council I helped to launch a comprehensive, two-pronged study to determine the availability, distribution, and utilization of primary health-care services in the London area. This study, the first of its kind, identified problems that the general public faced when attempting to find primary health care.[6] Later, in the spring of 1974, Edward Pickering, a retired Simpsons-

Sears executive, undertook an independent study of doctors for the Ontario Medical Association. He concluded, and I concurred, that better communication through publicly accessible education programs would benefit both doctors and patients. Pickering went on to explain that "Not only will the patient get the kind of response he feels he needs from his doctor, but in the process, the patient and the public will obtain a new understanding that doctors, after all, 'are humans too.'"[7]

These studies reflected many aspects of my philosophy of medical practice and community service. In my office waiting room, where patients were prohibited from smoking, I installed a small television set on which I played a looped video illustrating the effects of smoking. This video, which I had produced with the support of cardiologists, respiratory experts, and obstetricians, was graphic and to the point. Although its technical quality was primitive by contemporary standards, its content was compelling. In one segment a pregnant woman hooked up to an ultrasound machine is asked to smoke a cigarette. She inhales the smoke, and the ultrasound image shows the foetus in distress – it actually stops moving.[8] I played other in-house videos as well, and these focused on educating new parents about prenatal care and postpartum events. Firm in my belief that patients needed to understand not only the institutional procedures but also the medical protocol involved in obstetrics, I introduced a program of my own design to fill the gap. One evening a week I would screen a short film for expectant parents that covered prenatal care, what to expect during the mother's hospital stay, and postpartum care. Many of those who attended the screenings reported that the film and my willingness to answer all of their questions allowed them to relax and enjoy the miracle of bringing a new life into the world. Of course, some patients objected to my waiting room videos, saying that the information disturbed them. I told them that if they felt uncomfortable with what they had seen, then I had achieved a positive result. My staff also placed educational pamphlets and advertisements for community health-care programs in the waiting room. This was an innovative approach to assisting and educating patients, and it was foreign to many people's expectations of what should occur in a doctor's office.

As president of the London and District Academy of Medicine, which had a membership of 450, I worked with other like-minded medical practitioners to expand educational services. We found that many patient complaints arose because doctor and patient spoke on different levels; in consultation, they would skirt the patient's primary concerns without uncovering the true nature of the ailment. An informal member survey revealed that some patients had little or no idea what to expect during or after surgery, even in the case of minor procedures such as hernia repair or certain orthopaedic surgeries. It also came to light that many physicians felt uncomfortable with patients who had life-threatening diseases such as cancer. I believed that patients had the right to know as much about their condition as possible, although I did understand that many preferred not to know. Doctors had a responsibility to determine their patients' fundamental needs and desires.

Surveys also brought into focus the common patient complaint that doctors treat patients as though their illnesses are all in their heads, and I thought that this was worthy of further investigation. Reviewing the statistics, I discovered that 40 to 50 per cent of all conditions had a psychosomatic component, and this told me that people were experiencing more stress in their lives. Their pain was real, but its root cause had more to do with lifestyle pressures or personal habits than with an acute physical malady. If left untreated these people would suffer unnecessary pain and discomfort in their daily lives. As dedicated physicians we had to delve more deeply into our patients' lifestyle choices and activities in order to provide adequate treatment. For many of my colleagues this was a tall order. In my own practice I instructed office staff to listen carefully to each patient complaint, insisting that if the patient considered the situation an emergency, then it was an emergency. I told them to send such patients to the hospital emergency room, where I would meet them.

Many academy members agreed in theory to the need for expanded education programs, but a good number also argued, justifiably, that they already worked long hours, and active participation in such programs would cut into the little free time they had. Despite their reservations, I approached the academy's executive in early 1974 with a plan to create monthly public education forums; we would invite experts in various health-care fields to speak to lay and professional audiences. I also proposed implementing suggestions made in a Canadian nutrition study. This would involve putting together reports for the Ministry of Education and launching, at least at the district level, a thorough review of the nutritional value of school cafeteria meals. The academy also spearheaded more direct contact with the public in dealing with alcohol and drug abuse. Over the course of a decade most family physicians' offices, schools, factories, and institutions adopted elements of public health education, using pamphlets, posters, seminars, or films to reach out to men, women, and children from all walks of life. Like many initiatives, it took time and dedication, and I know that without the support of the academy, my colleagues, staff, family, and patients, I could not have poured so much into my role as public health educator.

Medical research continues to take quantum leaps. We are continually developing new drugs, treatments, procedures, and testing. When I was medical advisor to the Canadian Cancer Society, from 1972 to 1973, I learned of an inexpensive test, called the Hemoccult, for early detection of blood in the stool. Bleeding from the rectum is by no means an automatic indication of cancer – it can be caused by a variety of things, including hemorrhoids – but I saw this test as an invaluable tool because it allowed for early detection, diagnosis, and treatment of abnormal physical conditions of the colon and rectum. In the mid-1970s the test was still controversial, and many family physicians did not use it as part of their regular physical examinations. But, considering the dramatic reduction in cancer of the cervix brought about by the routine Pap smear, I decided to investigate this new method of early cancer detection. Although the Hemoccult test did not provide conclusive evidence of the presence or absence of bleeding and pathological changes, it would, I believed, help physicians to decide whether or not to order further tests.

After conducting further research on the test procedures and the supplies required, I began to screen all of my patients forty years and older for occult blood. In two years I administered the Hemoccult to over 2,000 patients, spotting thirty-two with cancer and thirty in a precancerous state.[9] (I sent the thirty with precancerous cells for further tests, such as sigmoidoscopies and barium enemas, and many years later, when I retired, all of these patients were healthy and enjoying their lives.) I shared my findings with colleagues at the Academy of Medicine and conferred with members of the College of Family Physicians, winning support from Dr John Sequin, the past president of the London chapter. He agreed that high-risk patients over the age of forty, especially males with a family history of bowel cancer, should be screened, and he noted that many doctors seemed apathetic towards employing the test on a routine basis. Moreover, few patients were even aware of the test. By 1977 only about 10 per cent of London's family physicians were offering the test to their patients. Obviously, more could be done to educate patients and doctors about this potentially life-saving test.

In January of 1978 I presented a paper on my survey results to the Pan-American Cancer Cytology Congress in Las Vegas. I told the audience that, guided by the results of Hemoccult testing, I had within two years reduced the incidence of invasive procedures (such as sigmoidoscopies) from 900 to 38.[10] In May 1979 I gave another paper on the subject, which included more statistical findings.

I made specific reference to other medical studies that supported my contention that the family doctor had a profound responsibility to incorporate preventative tests into routine physical examinations. Through these professional conferences and my work with the medical advisory committee for the Canadian Cancer Society, I was able to help increase public awareness. In March 1983 the *London Free Press* carried an article announcing the availability of free Hemoccult test kits for residents of London and the surrounding area. Every one of the city's 344 family physicians, internists, and gynecologists received one hundred test kits from the Canadian Cancer Society. The article also noted that London was "the first community in which the CR [colorectal] testing kits have been widely available. Described as a medical breakthrough, the CR tests proved to be as effective a diagnostic tool as the Pap smear, widely introduced in 1968."[11]

Throughout these years I appreciated those of my colleagues who supported me in my struggle to promote public health programs aimed at disease prevention. I shall always remember the words of Dr Mike Dillion, past president of the London and District Academy of Medicine, who described me as "a dedicated and responsible citizen of the community ... and almost a pioneer in the battle against smoking." He said these things during a 1984 awards ceremony when the academy presented me with the Glenn Sawyer Service Award, given "in recognition of an Ontario doctor's significant services to his profession and his community."[12] Most of the ceremony was a blur, but I remember feeling very close to the spirits of my mother and father and wishing that they could have been there with me on that special evening.

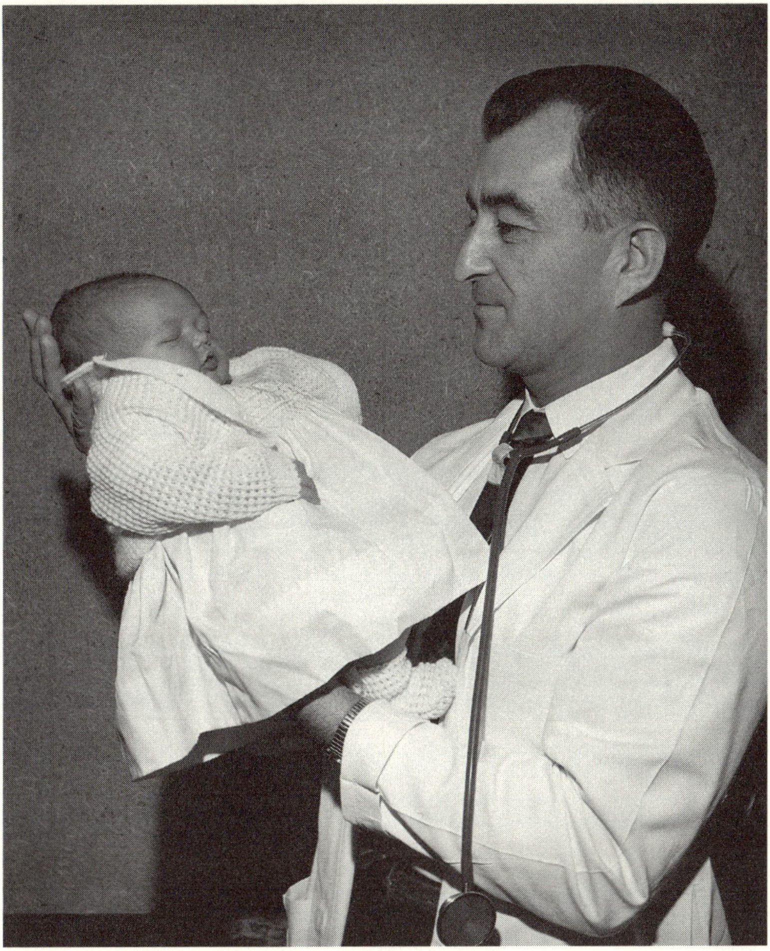

Boris holding London's centennial baby, born at 12:01 a.m., January 1967

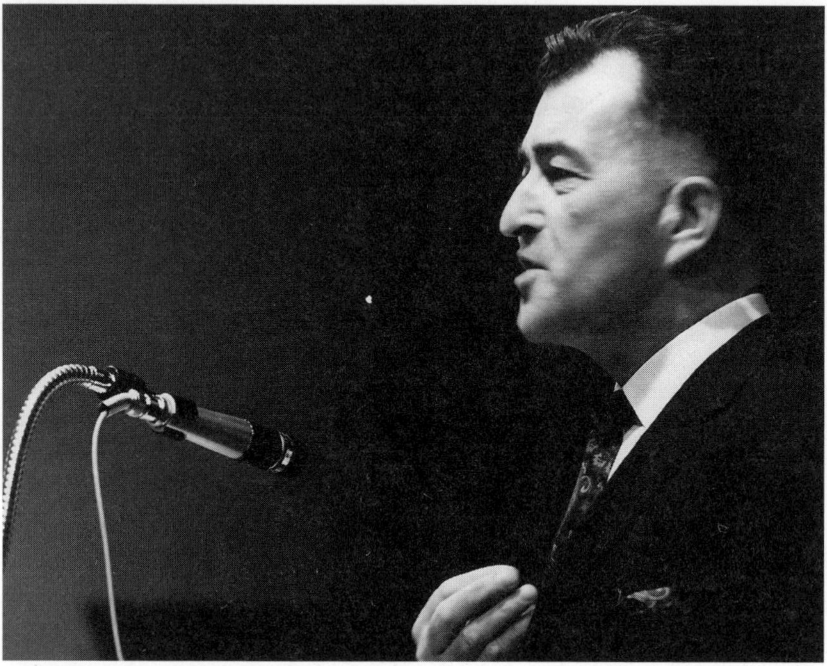

Boris addressing the London Chapter of the Academy of Medicine, c.1974

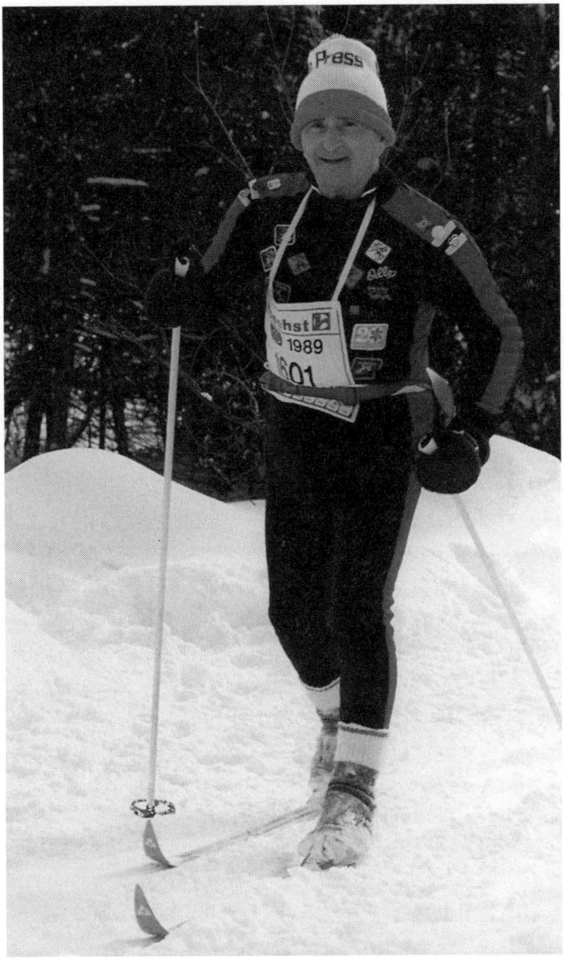

Boris participating in a two-day cross-country ski marathon from Montreal to Ottawa, 1989

8 I Believe in Miracles

I have always been a strong advocate of a healthy lifestyle. I made some mistakes, of course – like smoking cigarettes when I was younger – but for the most part I can truthfully say that I have always taken care of myself. As a prisoner of war I devised strategies, such as playing chess with myself and doing exercises, to maintain my psychological and physical health. However, as I approached middle age I had to juggle a busy medical practice and a thriving family, and finding the time to maintain physical fitness was a challenge. I decided to set aside one hour of the day – from 5:30 to 6:30 a.m. – for jogging, swimming, or cross-country skiing.

This personal lifestyle choice was of great benefit to me, and I began to think about how it could benefit my patients as well. My early research revealed that a daily exercise regime helped to fight a range of problems, such as obesity, coronary heart disease, hypertension, depression, and diabetes. Encouraging physical fitness also proved to be the most efficient and cost-effective approach to preventative medical care. I discussed these findings with my colleague Dr Joan Pivnick, and we pooled our resources and skills to introduce "the improved lifestyle and fitness concept ... to our patients."[1] We estimated that approximately 30 per cent of patients who made regular visits to their doctors could lessen the severity of their complaints by becoming more physically active, by avoiding smoking and excessive drinking, and by adopting better eating habits. In January 1980 a group of our patients willing to make positive changes entered the Fitness Ontario program, which was offered at the downtown London YM-YWCA.

Program director John Harrison evaluated every participant for such things as muscle strength, body fat, and respiratory function, and then fitness consultants designed individual exercise profiles based on physical condition. All participants received hands-on instruction in important training techniques, such as warming up and cooling down. Initially there were about fifty participants, but Joan and I, along with some other medical professionals, encouraged family physicians to recommend the fitness program to their patients, and the numbers climbed.

Joan and I were also in accord when it came to defining what the family physician's role and obligation to patients should be. Furthermore, we agreed that patients had to make a personal commitment to take charge of their lives and work towards improving their health. We circulated educational materials, which included information on breast-feeding and good nutrition. To decrease the likelihood of children developing food or other allergies later in life, Joan advised mothers to postpone giving their babies solid food until they were five months old. She also told them that breast milk (or a formula that is close to it) is best for babies of up to six months because it is easiest for them to digest and does not place unnecessary strain on their kidneys; moreover, breast milk, formula, and (later) homogenized milk provide babies with the fatty acids so essential to the healthy development of the brain.

As I mentioned earlier my ban on smoking in my office waiting room and similar policies and programs sometimes conflicted with my patients' views and expectations. I vividly recall one patient in his mid-forties who came for a checkup. He weighed in excess of 240 pounds and smoked three packs of cigarettes a day. Since he was a new patient I did a thorough examination, and I discovered that his blood pressure was 240 over 140 – dangerously high. His heart rate was normal, but a respiratory examination revealed that he was in the early stages of emphysema. In a forthright manner I explained to him that his addiction to smoking and his obesity exposed him to the risk of heart disease or stroke. When he asked me for a prescription to regulate his blood pressure I said, "I cannot give you a prescription unless you make a firm commitment to quit smoking, do daily exercise like walking, and reduce your weight by eating healthy foods." Glowering, he retorted, "So, you do not want to accept me as your patient?" I reiterated my conditions, and I explained that medication alone was not going to be of much help to him. In a fury he told me to "fuck off" and stormed out of the office. I sat quietly thinking over this encounter. In my heart I knew that I had been brutal and unbending, but I also knew that this patient could not be helped unless he was willing to help himself.

After a long and tiring day I wanted nothing more than my bed and sleep. I was awakened at about 11:00 p.m. by the ringing telephone. It was my angry patient. Before I could say a word he apologized for his behaviour and said, "Doctor, I decided to follow your advice. Will you take me on as a new patient?" I assured him that I would and told him to come to my office first thing in the morning to talk over the situation. He kept that appointment, and over the course of several months we were both gratified to see his blood pressure dropping. He quit smoking, although he hated having to go without his cigarettes. He started walking thirty minutes a day and changed his diet. Soon he had shed forty pounds. With some hard work this patient had stabilized his own condition, and he could now look forward to a much happier and healthier future. He later moved to the United States, and I lost touch with him. About two years after his departure he phoned to give me some exciting news. "Doctor," he announced, "you'll never believe this! I ran a marathon and finished in under five hours!" I was amazed and humbled. This man had helped to bring about a miracle.

Of course, I had long ago learned to practice what I preached – I'll never forget how embarrassed I was when the patient recovering from a heart attack admonished me for smoking at her bedside! So, with renewed determination I took up cross-country skiing, a sport I had loved as a child. In the summer I trained on roller skis, and once a year I competed in a two-day cross-country marathon from Montreal to Ottawa. More than 5,000 people participated in this event, and Ludmila often went with me to watch the skiers whoosh along the snowy trails. In all, I managed to compete twelve times. In my den at home I have several photographs that were taken of me at the start and finish lines, and they are not mere mementoes – they are tangible proof that one can achieve one's goals through hard work and persistence.

In principle making healthy lifestyle choices seemed simple enough, but I soon realized that many patients lacked both the time and the motivation. Life in burgeoning urban centres like London had become more complex. Many families now included two wage-earners. Work, child care, and the accelerated pace of life in general all made it difficult for many patients to maintain a healthy regime. In an attempt to reach out to these patients I organized a program at London's A.B. Lucas High School and invited everyone to join in. Participants not only learned about the benefits of exercises, but they also had fun – an important motivational force for many slow movers. The principal of the school was very impressed when he saw that program participants were developing better attitudes about healthy living. He regularly canvassed the high school students who took part, and he discovered that fully one-third of the non-addicted smokers had decided that cigarettes were a waste of time.

My work frequently inspired me to explore alternative methods of providing good medical care. One day an elderly patient who generally enjoyed good health came to my office complaining about her inability to sleep. As always I started to probe more deeply, asking her questions about her diet and any recent changes in her life. She was a devout Catholic, and she told me that her problems had started soon after Pope John XXIII had announced that the rosary was not essential for salvation. As I became attuned to her underlying distress, I asked her more questions, and she admitted that she had stopped praying with her rosary. I casually asked if she had her rosary with her, and she nodded. I encouraged her to relax and say her prayers; she did, and as I watched she entered a trance-like state. The woman seemed fully aware of where she was, but she had spiritually, or mentally, shifted to another level of consciousness. She appeared completely at peace. I had no medical explanation for her sleeplessness, and it dawned on me that her attachment to the rosary was central to the problem. I reassured my patient that the pope had not outlawed the use of the rosary and added that she should resume saying her prayers in the usual way. I also told her that I was confident she would be sleeping better soon and that she should see me again in a month's time. Relieved, she left the office. No, I had not prescribed a medicinal potion, but I had planted the idea in my patient's mind that she would be fine. And, yes, a month later she was happy to report that she no longer suffered from sleeplessness.

This patient taught me about the power of ideas and the capacity of the human mind to bring about positive change. I began researching hypnosis. I have always been open to alternative approaches to health care, refusing to discount the benefits of unproved therapies. If a patient believed that a copper bracelet could relieve arthritis pain, who was I to argue? We cannot know all there is to know in this world, but we can, and do, accept many phenomena on the basis of faith alone. Our ideas, formed and developed within the unknown realms of the mind, have the capacity to bring us peace and well-being.

In courses offered by the College of Family Physicians, I studied clinical hypnosis, earning a certificate from the Ontario division of the Canadian Society of Clinical Hypnosis in November 1990. As I gained confidence I began to use hypnosis to relieve my patients' pain and anxiety. One memorable day a mother brought in her two children, a boy and a girl, both under the age of six. The little boy had a smattering of warts on his hand, and, of course, his sister had contracted the same virus. Removing warts involves injections of a local anaesthetic and cauterisation, and I did not look forward to the howls of distress that this would induce. I asked the little fellow to climb up on the examination table. Holding his hand, I looked into his eyes and asked him about his favourite television shows. He told me that the funniest program was *The Flintstones*, and I asked him to pretend that he was watching it. The child went through the motions of turning on an imaginary television set. I asked him what Dino, the Flintstone family's pet dinosaur, was doing. As we proceeded with this game the boy would burst out laughing at the antics of the characters he was envisioning. At the same time I cauterized his warts. He remained completely absorbed in his "cartoon." Witnessing her brother's delight, the little girl clambered up beside him, insisting that she, too, liked *The Flintstones*. I had not used magic. Through hypnosis I had redirected the children's focus to a spectacle that they enjoyed.

Although I successfully applied hypnosis in my office for minor procedures, I remained unsure about using hypnoanaesthesia in surgical cases. But, once again, a patient's request for help provided me with the impetus and opportunity to hone new skills. I first met Jim, a family man in his mid-forties, when he came to see me about his addiction to tobacco and excessive drinking, and I treated him using hypnosis, positive reinforcement, and education. However, at one point he required hospitalization for emphysema. When I visited Jim on the ward he confided that he was worried about his future and that of his family. I assured him that if he made a real commitment to better lifestyle choices then he would get over this latest hurdle. "But Dr Ragula," he said, "there is something else. I have five children and I want a vasectomy." It was obvious that he had given this a lot of thought, so I explained the procedure to him and suggested that he have it done while he was still in the hospital. "That's fine," he responded, "but I want you to use hypnosis. I don't need anything else."

Although flattered by Jim's confidence in my abilities, I had some misgivings, and I wondered whether the hospital's surgery department would allow me to proceed. I was, finally, granted permission, but there would be an anaesthetist standing by in case Jim experienced any pain. On the day of the vasectomy several staff nurses and doctors joined us on the surgical ward. Jim seemed uneasy about this, but I induced a hypnotic state and he became oblivious to the onlookers. After the procedure he appeared relaxed, and he told me that he felt some tingling but no pain. Once Jim was settled comfortably in his hospital bed, staff members deluged me with questions. Many had never witnessed the application of hypnoanaesthesia; some said they viewed the technique as unconventional and perhaps unreliable. I did concede that this treatment method was not successful in all cases, but I was glad to note that some members of the medical staff managed to keep an open mind. I had seen so many medical professionals demonstrate a reluctance to accept new methods until shown documented proof of their efficacy. At every opportunity I would explain that with hypnosis patients voluntarily, with the help of a clinical practitioner, achieve an altered state of consciousness; hypnosis reduces and often eliminates the fear that causes tension and pain; and patients can emerge from this altered state whenever they wish, with the guidance of their practitioner.

One day Joan, a nurse at London's War Memorial Children's Hospital, came to my office. She was well aware of the range of childbirth methods available, but she was interested in trying hypnosis when it came time to have her own baby. A few years earlier I had introduced her to hypnosis when she needed relief from the pain of acute appendicitis. That positive experience coupled with her concerns about the effects of drugs, anaesthesia, and epidural injections on both mother and child convinced her that hypnosis offered a safer form of childbirth. We could use hypnosis to control Joan's uterine contractions, and it would afford me greater patient cooperation during the final stage of childbirth. By reducing physical shock and fatigue we could allow Joan a speedy recovery, and she would not have to contend with the post-operative effects of pain-killing drugs.

I asked Joan and her husband, Paul, to come to my office for training sessions. During the first session Joan sat in a reclining chair and gradually leaned back until she was comfortable. I asked her to visualize something pleasant – a person, place, or thing. She said that she would love to be on a sandy beach in Florida. By the time I had counted to five, Joan found herself on that beach. At one point I told her that she would feel contractions, but that these sensations would be pleasant because they were bringing her closer to the delivery of a healthy baby. The contractions, I suggested, were not going to be painful. After this we had several more sessions in which Joan learned to relax her face muscles, then her chest muscles, and so on. Most importantly, I cued Joan with the suggestion that whenever I or Paul placed our hands on her left shoulder she would relax and be able to control the contractions. Several times in the course of the training sessions Joan commented that while she knew what was happening to her she felt totally distanced from it all.

Two weeks before Joan's delivery date I admitted her to hospital because she had developed "leaky membranes" and I wanted her off her feet. I had intended to induce labour, but Joan's baby had other plans – she had decided that it was time to leave the womb. When I admitted Joan I instructed the attending staff to let my patient handle her delivery, but several nurses told her that they were worried because they had little experience with hypnosis. Joan replied that they had nothing to worry about, and if Dr Ragula did not arrive in time to help with the delivery then she knew they could manage. Joan's labour began at midnight, and when I arrived at the hospital the baby's head was already showing. After Joan gave birth to her daughter, Julie, the nurses questioned her about the experience. They had seen her go through labour with no sign of pain – she actually knitted between contractions! In the recovery room her uterus had come down quickly, and she produced breast milk earlier than usual. Some of the nurses expressed shock and disbelief when Joan got out of bed immediately after the birth and went to the bathroom, took a shower, and walked down the hall to the nursery. Everyone was prepared for her to faint, but she remained in control and everything was fine.[2]

I often relied on scientific methods and research to help me develop programs and treatments for my patients. However, I also admit quite freely that I have accepted that miracles do happen. For me, the most wonderful miracle is childbirth. Science intervenes and presents us with measurements of fetal development, yet there is still an element of the divine in the birth of a child. I marvelled at the miracle of my own children's births, and when I helped to deliver my patients' children I was always overwhelmed and elated upon hearing the baby's first cries.

My only daughter, Rahnieda, and I share the same birthday – 1 January. Because of my busy practice it often happened that we could not spend our special day together. On 31 December 1966 Rahnieda lamented this fact, and I promise to do everything I could to celebrate this birthday with her. However, St Joseph's called in the early afternoon to tell me that one of my patients had been admitted in the early stages of labour. I decided to say nothing to Rahnieda at this point. At 10:00 p.m. the hospital called again to inform me that my patient was now in active labour. By 11:45 p.m. I was scrubbed and my patient was in the last stages of delivery. Emily, a beautiful baby girl, came into the world at one minute past midnight. She was London's celebrated "centennial baby," and her timely arrival allowed me to spend 1 January 1967 with my own precious daughter.

Emily's parents divorced and left London some years after her birth, and I lost touch with the family. Seventeen years later a lovely young woman came to my office and coyly asked if I recognized her. When I told her that I did not she said, "Well, you should. You were the first man in my life." Taken aback, I wondered what the implications of her announcement could be. Then she pointed to the picture of the centennial baby hanging on my wall and said, "That's me – your centennial baby." Emily had a gentle and teasing sense of humour, and I was very pleased (and relieved) to learn that she had come to ask me to be her family doctor. A few years later, after she had married and become pregnant, she asked me to deliver her baby. By this time I had given up obstetrical work, not because I wanted to, but because I was now nearing retirement and I thought that younger doctors could handle deliveries better than I. But Emily was very insistent, so I applied for a one-day hospital privilege to deliver her baby. I was once again allowed to share in the miracle of childbirth.

As the years went by I found that the needs of my long-time patients were changing. Married couples who had raised families and retired from their occupations demonstrated a variety of stress-related symptoms. Many of these people had not prepared for their "golden years," and they were encountering marital problems. It fell to me to counsel these troubled patients and help them to come to terms with their dramatically changed lives. I remember one couple who were adamant that they wanted to divorce after more than forty years together. Despite my best efforts, they could not overcome their personal rift. After giving their case much thought I presented them with pencil and paper and placed a calculator on my desk. Then I told them that this would be our last counselling session because they had considered many alternatives and divorce seemed inevitable. However, I continued, I wanted their indulgence. I asked them to list all of their assets, income, and investments. Once they had completed this exercise I had them itemize the costs they would incur if they lived apart. Two apartment rents, two telephone bills, two cars, and so on. Fingers flying, I added up the damage on the calculator and showed them that divorce would drastically alter their standard of living. As they left my office I thought I noted a subtle change in their attitude towards one another. About a month later they reported to me that they had decided to stay married after all. Moreover, they had made a concerted effort to overlook one another's irritating habits, which had initially created the disharmony. They were also volunteering in the community and had joined several clubs. It seemed that all they had really needed was a little push, and I was happy to have provided it for them.

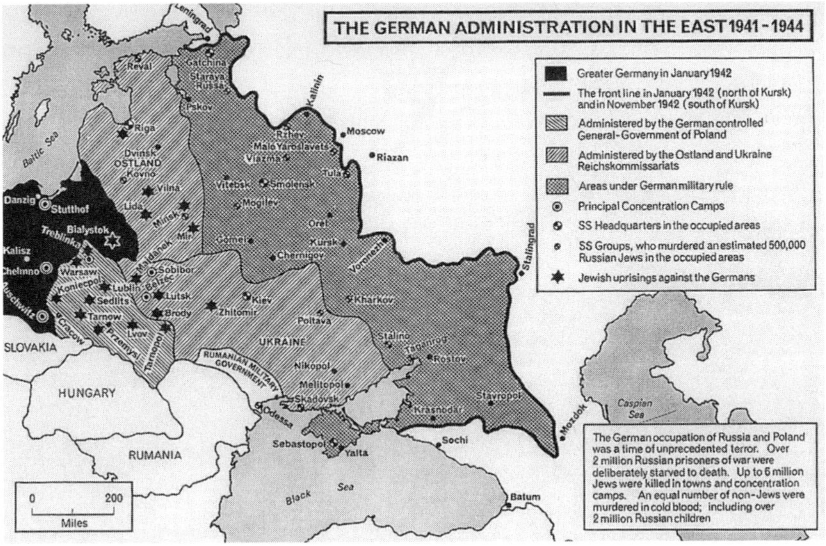

The German Administration in the East, 1941–44

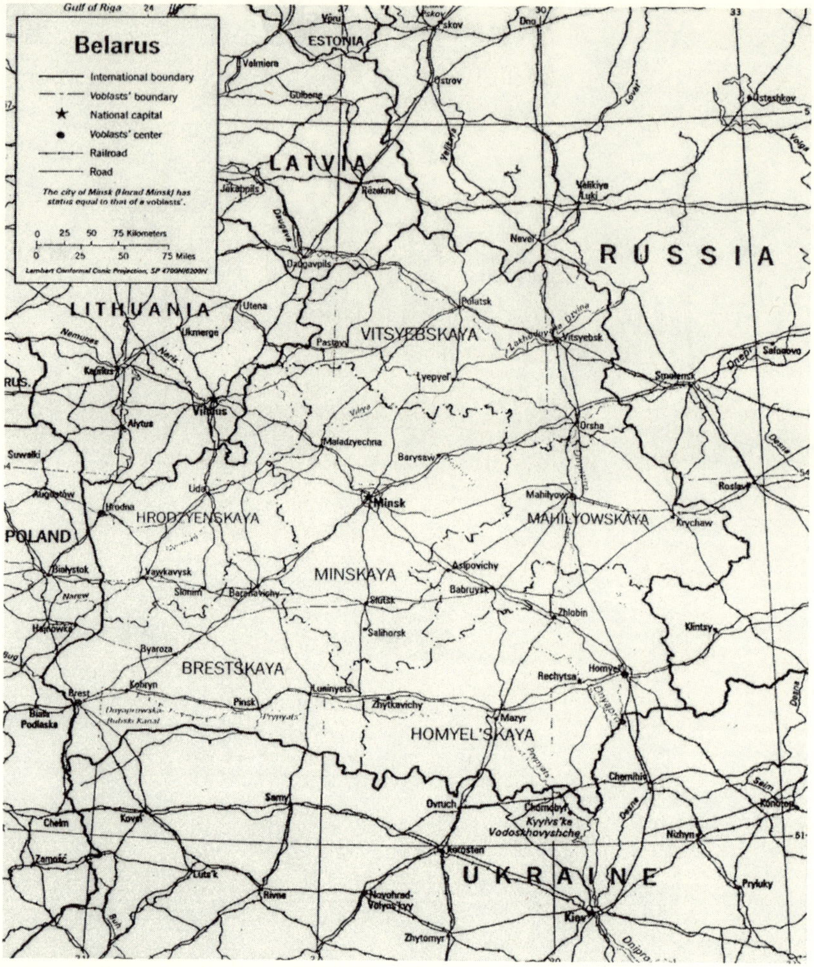

Map of Belarus, 1997, courtesy of the Sauer Map Library, University of Western Ontario

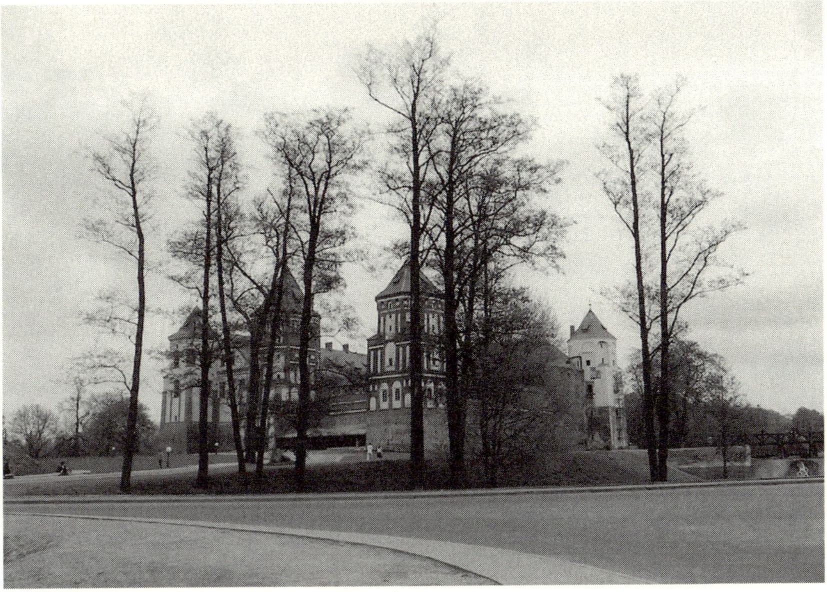

Mir Castle, courtesy of Sandra Hobson. The castle, an architectural monument dating from 1495, sustained heavy damage over the centuries; today it is being restored to its former glory

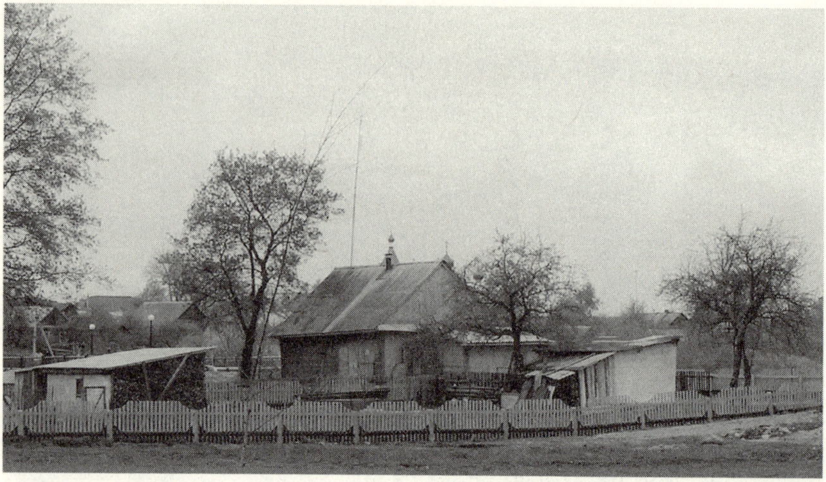

A typical village in rural Belarus, near Mir Castle, courtesy of Sandra Hobson

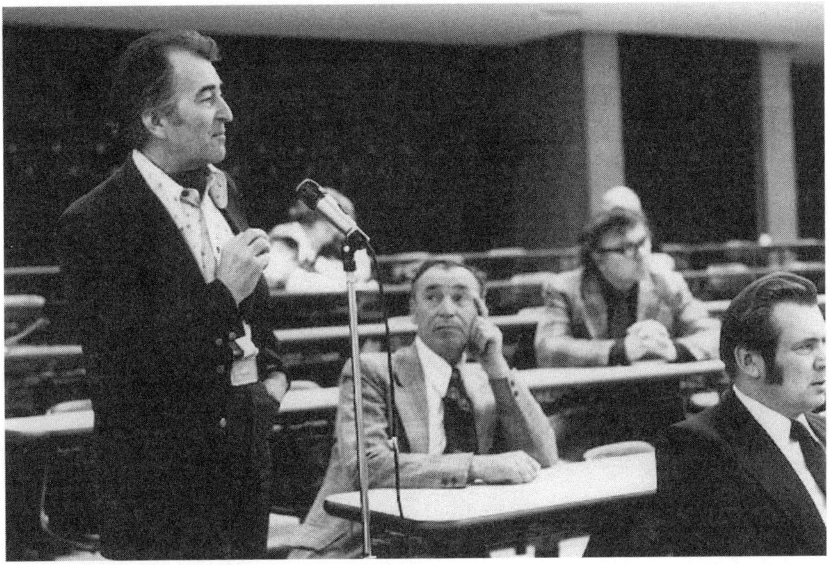

Boris at the Belarusian Institute of Arts and Sciences, Ottawa, 1975, courtesy of Joanna Survilla

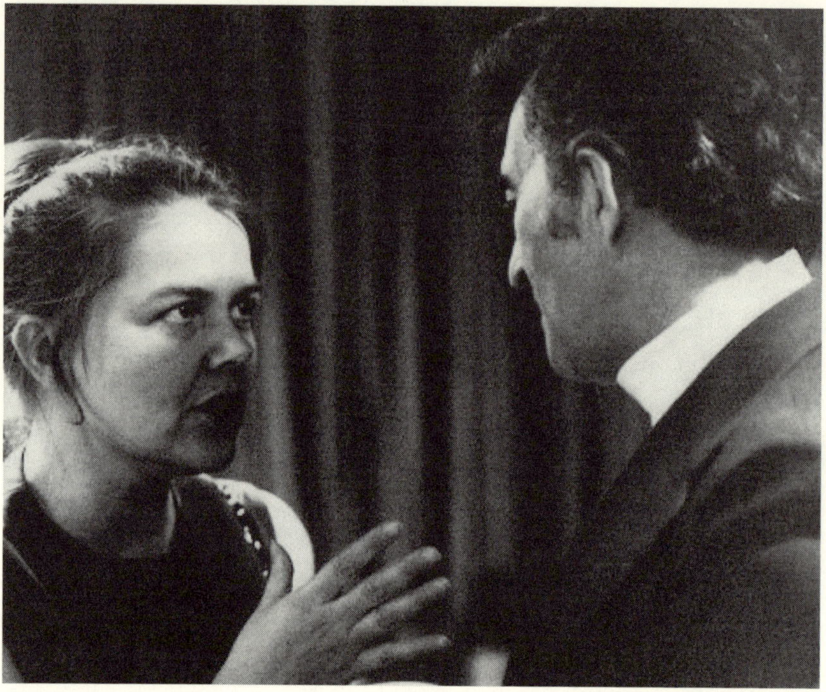

Boris with Joanna Survilla, 1975, courtesy of Joanna Survilla.

Epilogue

Eastern Europeans and others saw their idealistic aspirations to maintain territorial integrity, cultural identity, and religious and linguistic self-determination trampled by the forces of German Nazism and Soviet totalitarianism. Stalin's reign of terror and World War II created political and social upheaval in Belarus and elsewhere in Europe. Through his stories Boris Ragula offers us a personal perspective of these important events.

Perhaps better than most people, Boris accepts the limits of mortal time. One cannot help but marvel at the fact that he survived a German POW camp, a NKVD death camp, and torture; he found love, he fought for his ideals, and he grasped every available opportunity. Communism, as constructed by Stalin and his followers, robbed millions of men, women, and children of their freedom of speech and their freedom to live out their lives. Boris fought Communism's terrible effects through philanthropy and his involvement in organizations that provided aid to his beloved homeland.

When the explosion tore apart reactor number 4 at the Chernobyl Nuclear Power Station on 26 April 1986, Belarusians living abroad were galvanized into action, aiding their homeland as never before, and Boris Ragula was among them. Prior to the Chernobyl disaster Boris had made regular contributions to charities that aided Belarusians at home and abroad. He had also participated in the Rada of the Belarusian National Congress, an organization dedicated to providing aid to Belarusians and to reinforcing the ideals of social and cultural self-determination and political autonomy. Boris, and other like-minded Belarusians, never forgot that in 1918 Belarus had become the Belarusian Democratic Republic under the leadership of liberals who worked to organize a new order after the collapse of the Russian tsarist regime. This new government soon found itself forced into exile by the Soviet military powers, and many of those involved in the formation of a democratic Belarus took refuge in Prague. The current Rada of the Belarusian National Republic is headquartered in New York City, and it sees itself as the spiritual heir of the 1918 Rada.

The 1986 Chernobyl disaster was compounded by an event that illustrated the democratic promise of Belarus and the limitations that would soon be imposed. On 3 June 1988 the Belarusian journal *Literature and Art* published a detailed report on the notorious Kuropaty Forest on the northeast edge of Minsk, claiming that an estimated 300,000 bodies were buried in mass graves there. All were victims of Stalin's reign of terror against Belarus during the period 1937–40; Boris clearly remembers being threatened by the NKVD with execution and burial in Kuropaty. Despite official attempts to discredit the discoveries, the Belarusian Popular Front, organized in 1988, pressured the government to maintain the momentum of an unofficial investigation of Kuropaty. The Popular Front, which had many university lecturers among its members, was eventually targeted by the Belarusian government, and the organization's newspapers, meetings, and demonstrations were banned.

Nonetheless, Belarusian nationalists had found their voice, and large numbers of them became founding members of the Charitable Fund for the Children of Chernobyl. The project encouraged people and organizations in foreign countries to send aid to children in the Chernobyl zone and arrange for them to visit abroad. Boris and his fellow Belarusians living abroad believed that by helping these children Belarusians would bolster their efforts to help themselves following the Chernobyl explosion and the subsequent breakup of the Soviet Union.

Boris became a member of the Rada and served as its president from 1996 to 1998. Rada members believed that they could contribute to a political awakening and create the impetus for change in Belarus. Events buoyed their expectations. When the Soviet Union collapsed in 1991 the leaders of three East Slavic Soviet socialist republics – Boris Yeltsin of Russia, Leonid Kuchma of Ukraine, and Stanislav Shushkevich of Belarus – met at a hunting lodge in the Belovezhskaya Pushcha (the Belarusian Forest) in December 1991. The leaders proclaimed the end of the USSR and the inauguration of three independent countries, which would comprise the Commonwealth of Independent States. They invited other former Soviet republics to join them. Boris and his Belarusian friends abroad believed that they were witnessing the dawn of a new, democratic era.

Boris held that Belarusians now had an opportunity to move towards the liberal and democratic goals inspired by the leaders of the 1918 Rada. He attended meetings of the Rada in North America and Europe; he developed contacts among Belarusian politicians; and he broadcast democratic messages to Belarusians from Prague. However, within a few years it became apparent that Belarus was failing to achieve political and social autonomy. Liberal and democratic hopes diminished after the first election following the collapse of the USSR. In 1992, marking the first free election in the history of Belarus, Shushkevich – a physicist from the Belarusian State University who had also served as chairman of the Supreme Soviet – lost to Aleksandr Lukashenko, a populist politician and former collective-farm chairman. Lukashenko used his position as chairman of the parliamentary anti-corruption committee to mount a vicious attack on Shushkevich, knowing that rural voters would prefer a conservative, authoritarian president who espoused a political order similar to the old Soviet system of governance.

Once elected, Lukashenko, with the support of a tame Parliament, imposed a series of political changes on Belarus that clearly resembled Soviet totalitarianism. Belarusians living abroad were deflated when the population of their homeland elected Lukashenko and endorsed a renewed Stalinist order. Domestic and foreign observers questioned the election results during the period 1994–96. In the November 1996 election skeptics observed many irregularities, and they challenged the validity of Lukashenko's victory at the polls. Still, Lukashenko enjoyed the support of an elderly, cautious peasant population wedded to the ways they had learned under decades of Communist rule.

Boris, while discouraged by the election outcome and subsequent political developments in Belarus, continued to help others through various philanthropic undertakings. In 1990 he joined Joanna Survilla of the Belarusian Institute of Arts and Sciences, Canada; Zina Gimpelevich of the University of Waterloo; and several others to found the Canadian Relief Fund for Chernobyl Victims in Belarus, which, in turn, worked with the Charitable Fund, Children of Chernobyl, in Minsk. Through this program, Canadian host families brought children from Chernobyl to London and other participating centres in Canada. These visits gave the children a respite from their impoverished, possibly contaminated, environment, and the opportunity to receive eyeglasses, dental work, and instruction in dental hygiene and healthy eating habits. Since the program was launched several hundred Belarusian children have spent six weeks in Canada, and many have returned at the special invitation of their host families for annual visits. While he was still practising Boris attended to the minor medical problems of these Belarusian children. He and Ludmila also invited those suffering from homesickness to spend a few days with them – at the Ragula home they enjoyed familiar Belarusian food and conversation in their own language around the kitchen table.

In 1992 Boris, with the support of Dr G.Z. Wright of the University of Western Ontario's Faculty of Medicine and Dentistry, chaired a fundraising committee for Operation Belarus, an initiative launched by Western to establish professional interaction between London-based paediatric dentists and the children's dental clinic at Minsk Medical Institute. Over time the program upgraded the clinic's dental technology and improved the training of Belarusian dentists. Appealing to Belarusians in Canada, the United States, Australia, and Great Britain, Boris raised $30,000 for dental equipment for the Minsk clinic – six fully equipped dental stations were purchased.

Boris also initiated a doctors' program under the auspices of the Canadian Relief Fund and later turned the supervision of the program over to Charles Ruud, a professor of Russian history at Western and an active member of the fund's London chapter. Through this project at least one Belarusian medical doctor is invited each year to spend several weeks in Canada to observe current medical practices. The project was important to Boris because he knew that Canadian medical specialists who had interacted with Belarusian doctors and dentists in Canada and in Belarus had noted problems with Belarusian medical education and practice. The Belarusian doctors desperately needed new medical equipment if they were to implement up-to-date medical ideas and techniques. Moreover, their medical schools had a pressing need for access to medical journals and the Internet.

With strong support from Western's Faculty of Medicine and Dentistry, the London Health Sciences Centre, and the Belarusian

State Medical University, a team of Canadian doctors, nurses, radiologists, and occupational therapists make annual ten-day visits to Minsk. Charles Ruud has organized and led these visits, escorting specialists in cardiology, ophthalmology, and neurology, among other fields, on exchanges between the University of Western Ontario and institutions in Belarus. Belarusian medical authorities declare that the exchange has had an enormous positive impact on Belarusian medical practice and the general health of the people. Also, medical supply companies have worked with the London chapter of the Canadian Relief Fund to ship over two million dollars' worth of medical equipment, devices, and medicines to Belarus. Characteristically, Boris Ragula insists that he has played only a small part in all of these humanitarian efforts.

To a certain degree advancing age dictated a slower pace of life for Boris, but his faith in the ideal of a democratic Belarus remained strong, and he continued to give generously to organizations that aid Belarus. He passed his Rada presidency on to Joanna Survilla at the end of his term. Through his recollections Boris inspired people of all ages to hold on to their dreams and delve deeply into their hearts and minds to find the strength of will they will need to achieve their personal goals. "Every one of us has untapped powers, untapped resources," Boris once remarked, "and when one believes this, then miracles can happen. People can control their own destinies."

After each of my visits with Boris, I left him sitting in a quiet reverie, for as he spoke a lifetime of memories would come flooding back. In this memoir we encounter a remarkable man who possessed a rare combination of compassion and steely determination, a man with the heart of a rebel who imagined the possible and sought to make it a reality.

Boris Ragula passed away on 21 April 2005.

Inge Sanmiya
30 April 2005

Notes

CHAPTER ONE

1 Helen Fedor, ed., *Belarus*, Library of Congress Country Studies (Washington: Library of Congress, June 1995).
2 "Jogaila" is also written as "Jagiello."
3 Paul Robert Magocsi, *Historical Atlas of East Central Europe* (Seattle and Washington: University of Washington Press, 1993), 71.
4 Ibid. The February Revolution and the Bolshevik Revolution threw the Russian empire into turmoil. Belarusians had little sympathy for the Bolsheviks. Instead, the Socialist Revolutionary Party; the Mensheviks, a group advocating parliamentary, gradual socialism rather than the violent overthrow promoted by the Bolsheviks; the Bund, a Jewish Socialist movement; and a variety of Christian movements dominated Belarus's burgeoning political life.

5 This practice of informing on the citizenry had been imposed on the Orthodox Church by the Spiritual Regulations of Peter I in 1721.

CHAPTER TWO

1 In December 1917 the first Soviet state security organization was created. The Vecheka (All-Russian Extraordinary Commission for Combatting Counter-Revolution and Sabotage) was more commonly known as the Cheka. The following year the NKVD (People's Commissariat of Internal Affairs) was formed to control the militia (police), criminal-investigation departments, fire brigades, internal troops, and prison guards. In March 1946 the Soviet government was restructured, and all people's commissariats were designated ministries – thus the NKVD became the MVD. On 13 March 1954 the reformed MVD was permitted to retain its traditional policing and internal security functions, while the new KGB took on state security functions. The KGB was subordinated to the USSR Council of Ministers, the Soviet Cabinet of that time.

2 I know now that the place Ginsberg referred to was Kuropaty, a wooded area not far from Minsk. Thousands of Belarusians were executed there for crimes they did not commit. It was not until 1988 that the authorities discovered mass graves at Kuropaty containing the remains of over 30,000 victims. Each had been shot once in the head.

CHAPTER THREE

1 See Michael R. Marrus, *The Holocaust in History* (London: Penguin Books, 1987), 71–83. Marrus discusses how the Germans relied heavily "upon native police and administrative personnel. While the degree of cooperation varied, it existed practically everywhere." Moreover, in every occupied country, Germans enlisted "legions of helpers: in governments, ministries, police, private industries, and the railways" (83).

2 Green, red, and white were the national colours of Belarus.

CHAPTER FOUR

1 The Polish representative was stationed in London, England, but he was in Vilnius in 1944 to try to establish formal alliances between Poland and Belarus.

2 Some time after I arrived in Germany, I did find Rudy's mother, and I gave her Rudy's message. She clung to me, crying and saying that she had always believed Rudy was a good boy and a good German.

CHAPTER FIVE

1 See Nikolai Tolstoy, *Victims of Yalta* (London: Hodder and Stoughton, 1977), for more information on the repatriation activities of British and American authorities. Belarusians living outside the Soviet Union feared reprisals from the Stalinist state and felt powerless when attempting to explain their concerns to representatives of the Allied Forces. On many occasions we relied on unofficial or black market sources to provide us with the travel documents we needed to escape, once again, the shroud of Communist rule.

2 In the immediate post-war period, events in Eastern Europe provoked bitter conflicts among the former allies. At the Yalta Conference, American and British diplomats – among them President Franklin Roosevelt – had agreed to recognize the Soviet sphere of influence in the border region occupied by the Red Army. It soon became apparent that the Soviets had no intention of allowing free elections or permitting democratic political parties to exist. In 1946, in Fulton, Missouri, Winston Churchill delivered the famous policy speech in which he warned, "From Strettin in the Baltic to Trieste in the Adriatic, an Iron Curtain has descended across the continent."

3 For 321 days American planes flew more than 270,000 missions to bring food and supplies to Berlin after the Soviet Union had blocked all surface routes to the city. The blockade was finally lifted on 12 May 1949. In October of that year the Soviet Union had created a separate government for East Germany, which became the German Democratic Republic.

4 Rahneida was named after the Belarusian princess who brought Christianity to Belarus in the tenth century; Vitaut was named after a prince of ancient Belarus. We gave our children these names because we wanted to keep a part of our past and our future with us always.

5 I had also received offers to work in Windsor, Ontario, and a small community in northern Ontario, but my professor suggested London.

6 Walter now resides in the United States, and we are still close friends.

CHAPTER SIX

1 I bought a small life insurance policy and named Michael Ragula as the beneficiary to give my cousin collateral assurance for this substantial loan. Looking back I also realize that I wanted to demonstrate to my colleagues, friends, and family that I was taking responsibility for my family's future. Perhaps I was motivated by pride, but by adopting a business-like approach to Michael's loan I was also avoiding family money squabbles.

2 "Grandmother Gives Man a Kidney," *London Free Press*, 31 March 1964. See also "London Transplant: Grandmother's Kidney Keeps Man, 21, Alive," *Globe and Mail*, 31 March 1964. In September 1963 the same team – Callaghan, Reese, and Carroll – had transplanted a kidney from a cadaver into the body of a male patient. The patient died a week later.

3 D and C is used to control sudden, heavy vaginal bleeding, which causes a decrease in blood volume or the number of red blood cells. The procedure involves passing a small instrument, called a curette, through the vagina into the uterus and scraping the endometrium – the lining of the uterus. It is the quickest way to stop uterine bleeding. D and C is also used to obtain tissue samples for testing older women who have a high risk of developing endometrial cancer.

4 The Papanicolaou Vaginal Smear, also called the Pap smear, was devised by Dr George N. Papanicolaou, who emigrated to the United States from Greece in 1917 and worked at the Pathology Department of Cornell Medical College. Prompted by his wife's sterility, he started

to study vaginal smears, and he noticed a variation in the appearance of vaginal cells in relation to ovulation. By 1921 Papanicolaou was able to refine his technique and positively identify abnormal cells, which, after a biopsy, confirmed the presence of cervical cancer.

5 Two other journals accepted articles I wrote on Pap smears and early detection: *Canadian Family Physician* (October 1967 and June 1968) and *Cancer Cytology* (June 1968).

CHAPTER SEVEN

1 "Shock Treatment: Doctors Quit Smoking after Getting a Look at What It Does," *London Free Press*, 22 September 1971.

2 Ibid. Auerbach met with criticism from all quarters. Many denounced his work as invalid because his subjects were dogs, not human beings. He suspected that a great deal of the criticism had been initiated by tobacco lobbyists.

3 While the OMA was, and still is, a voluntary organization, and its decisions are not enforceable by law, it represented the province's 14,000 physicians and its pronouncements did have an impact on public and professional opinion.

4 "OMA Backs Local Body's Stand, Labels Doctors' Smoking 'Improper,'" *London Free Press*, 29 May 1974.

5 "Rules for Non-smoking Rated as Unacceptable," *London Free Press*, 10 January 1977.

6 "Study of Primary Health Care Services," *London Free Press*, 18 December 1973. The study defined primary health care as the first component of the health-services system that a person in need of attention comes in contact with. The primary health-care supplier could be a hospital emergency room nurse, a physician, a social worker, or a public health nurse. Dr Ian McWhinney, chairman of the division of family medicine in the Department of Community Medicine at the University of Western Ontario, co-ordinated the study.

7 "London Academy of Medicine President Seeking to Open Two-Way Street of Candour," *London Free Press*, 19 March 1974.

8 One pregnant patient of mine threw away her cigarettes right after she saw the video. This bright and articulate woman had been unaware

of the threat to her unborn child until she was presented with the graphic evidence of the recorded ultrasound.

9 See Boris Ragula, "Regular Screening Would Reduce Cancer of Colon and Rectum Toll," *Journal of the American Medical Association*, 13 October 1975. The Hemoccult test was introduced in 1970 by SmithKline Diagnostics of Sunnyvale, California. On three consecutive days – because gastrointestinal bleeding may be intermittent – the patient smears fecal samples with a wooden applicator on a guaiac-impregnated paper slide.

10 Anoscopy, proctoscopy, and sigmoidoscopy tests allow a doctor to examine the anus, rectum, and lower part of the large intestine (colon) for abnormal growths such as tumours or polyps, bleeding, hemorrhoids, and conditions such as diverticulosis. All of these tests are performed by inserting viewing instruments into the anus, rectum, or colon. A barium enema is a test that allows the doctor to examine the large intestine (colon). A whitish liquid (barium) is introduced through the rectum into the colon and large intestine; the barium outlines the inside of the colon so that it can be seen more clearly on an X-ray. This test is often used to determine the cause of rectal bleeding or blood in the stool; it may help detect diseases such as inflammatory bowel disease or diverticulosis; and it can be employed as a diagnostic tool in the early detection of colon cancer.

11 "Free Testing Kits to Detect Colon-Rectal Cancer Available," *London Free Press*, 26 March 1983.

12 "Work in Public Health Programs Brings Special Medical Award," *London Free Press*, 29 June 1984.

CHAPTER EIGHT

1 "Doctor Prescribing Fitness for His Patients," *London Free Press*, 31 March 1980. Joan Pivnick joined my practice in the early 1980s, soon after she had completed her internship at St Joseph's Hospital. She later married and moved to the United States.

2 See Pamela J. Keddie, "Hypnoanaesthesia in Childbirth," *Great Expectations*, summer 1982. This parenting magazine article gives

a detailed account of Joan's training and childbirth experience. Joan was dedicated to the training and achieved autohypnosis, but some patients cannot do this, and they require a trained hypnotherapist to be present during the delivery. And even patients who have achieved an altered state may be rocketed out of it by the screams of patients in adjoining labour-room cubicles.

Suggested Further Reading

Andreas, Peter, and Timothy Snyder, eds. *The Wall around the West: State Borders and Immigration Controls in North America and Europe.* Lanham, MD: Rowman and Littlefield, 2000.

Bernier, Jacques. *Disease, Medicine and Society in Canada: A Historical Overview.* Ottawa: Canadian Historical Association, 2003.

Bertsch, Gary K. *Reform and Revolution in Communist Systems: An Introduction.* New York: Macmillan, 1991.

Coburn, David, Carl D'Arcy, and George M. Torrance, eds. *Health and Canadian Society: Sociological Perspectives.* Toronto: University of Toronto Press, 1998.

Hoerder, Dirk. *Creating Societies: Immigrant Lives in Canada.* McGill-Queen's Studies in Ethnic History 2.5. Montreal and Kingston: McGill-Queen's University Press, 1999.

Igoa, Cristina. *The Inner World of the Immigrant Child*. New York: St. Martin's Press, 1995.

Kennedy, Paul, and Victor Roudometof, eds. *Communities across Borders: New Immigrants and Transnational Cultures*. London and New York: Routledge, 2002.

Marples, David R. *Belarus: A Denationalized Nation*. Amsterdam: Harwood Academic, 1999.

Quack, Sybil, ed. *Between Sorrow and Strength: Women Refugees and the Nazi Period*. New York: German Historical Institute, 1995.

Spencer, Hanna. *Hanna's Diary, 1938–1941: Czechoslovakia to Canada*. Montreal and Kingston: McGill-Queen's University Press, 2001.

Tan, Amy. *The Bonesetter's Daughter*. New York: Putnam, 2001.

Zaprudnik, Jan. *Belarus: At a Crossroads in History*. Boulder, CO: Westview Press, 1993.

Index